# HOW TO STOP OVERTHINKING WOMEN EDITION

Reduce negative thoughts and Anxiety

# TABLE OF CONTENTS

# INTRODUCTION

It is effortless to fall into the device of overthinking about minor things throughout everyday life. So, when you are contemplating something, pose necessary inquiries to yourself. It has been found through an exploration that extending the viewpoint by utilizing these straightforward inquiries can snap you rapidly out of overthinking.

Endeavor to set brief time-limits for choices. So, figure out how to turn out to be better at settling on opportunities and to get a move on setting due dates in your everyday life. Regardless of when it is a little or a more excellent choice.

Be a person of movement. When you understand how in the first place making a move dependably, then you will wait less by overthinking. Setting due dates is one thing that will assist you with being a person of activity.

Endeavor to acknowledge one significant thing that you can't control everything. Attempting to thoroughly consider a thing multiple times can be an approach to endeavor to control everything, so you don't hazard committing an error, fall flat or resembling a trick. Those things are a piece of carrying on with a real existence where you genuinely extend your usual range of familiarity.

State stop in a condition where you understand you can't think straight. Now and again, when you are avaricious or when you are lying in bed and are going to rest, by the negative thoughts start murmuring around in your mind.

Do whatever it takes not to wind up stirred up in vague feelings of trepidation. Another snare that you have fallen into ordinarily that have impelled on overthinking is that you have lost all sense of direction in dubious feelings of fear about a circumstance in your life. Thus, your mind running wild has made fiasco situations about what could occur if you accomplish something. What is the most terrible that could happen? You ought to figure out how to pose this inquiry to yourself.

Invest the vast majority of your energy right now. Be right now in your regular day to day existence instead of before or a conceivable future. Hinder how you do whatever you are doing well at this point. Move slower, talk slower, or ride your bike all the more gradually, for instance. By doing as such, you become increasingly mindful of how you utilize your body and what's going on surrounding you at present.

Endeavor to invest the more significant part of your energy with individuals who don't think more. Your social condition has considerable influence. Discover approaches to spend the more substantial portion of your energy and consideration with the general population and sources that effects affect your reasoning.

# CHAPTER ONE
## Countering Overthinking: Step Towards an Improved Life

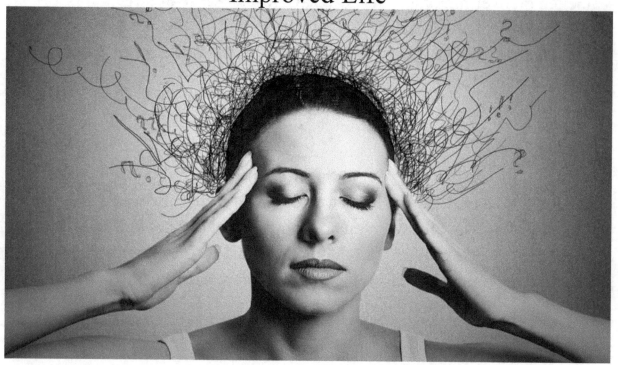

So, suppose you're hanging about at a social event, encompassed by partners and customers, and you have spotted somebody you genuinely need to converse with. Perhaps its business related, or you need to develop personal ties. How it is, you set up a psychological draft of what to state, as one does, and mean to meet them however a shivering apprehension in the back of your head leaves you speechless. Consider the possibility that they would prefer not to chat with you. Imagine a scenario where the specific line of discussion doesn't work out. Or then again even turns out badly? Your dread makes a kind of domino impact, and you start to think about the most terrible that could occur as the inescapable. With each idea, you are maneuvered further into the tangled wreckage of perplexity inside your psyche, and this, eventually, renders you unfit to try and talk any longer. You at that point, watch as someone else engages in discussion with the subject: an open door lost.

Overthinking and the resulting fretfulness and tension, while demonstrates to be a considerable hindrance in one's social and personal life, is additionally shockingly normal and for each person who is an injured individual to it, turns into the reason for circumstances lost and minutes that one would later lament. In any case, with a couple of day by day rehearses and a decoded frame of mind, it tends to be defeated effectively.

## Acknowledgment

The initial move towards managing intemperate overthinking and tension is tolerating the issue in any case. Directly after this, would you have the option to feel free to settle it? In any case, while realizing that you are a remunerator is significant, it is likewise indispensable that you understand that you are not the only one in the circumstance and that there is no motivation to freeze. Overthinking is a common thing among many individuals today, and you would almost certainly beat it with an inspirational demeanor.

## The best minute is the present minute.

The best thing you can do about overthinking is clearly to remain with the present. Your cerebrum can't consider faraway issues if it's bustling where it ought to be with the stream. You additionally figure out how to value your environment, and being in the present improves your presentation on any assignment fundamentally. Also, even though it is a lot more complicated than one might expect, there are a couple of strategies which you can practice day by day to limit the cycle of negative musings as it were.

One good precedent is relaxing. You'd be shocked at how much this makes a difference. Close your eyes and take full breaths for several minutes. Intently watching and taking full breaths help to pull you in the present minute, and helps in clearing your head.

Another good precedent is reflecting on rehearsing care. The essential thought is to stay quiet and just spotlight on all that is around you intently, and this has done some incredible things for many individuals. Just once every day, close your eyes and attempt to take in the entirety of your environment. Tune in to your considerations; however, don't 'connect' with them, and inevitably, you can try to cut back their 'volume.'

Notwithstanding that, back off. Do all that you do with full consciousness of you doing it. Attempt and describe to yourself each progression that you make, and power yourself to see your environment. This will likewise assist you with staying right now.

**Be certain**

At the point when full to the overflow with confidence and liking yourself, you develop a positive outlook. You would end up to be less inclined to overthinking; thus, everything that you do or say ends up being improved. First things you can do is get occupied. Structure an arrangement of what to accomplish for the afternoon, and continue being profitable. Doing things shield your brain from straying, and notwithstanding that, completing stuff results in an extraordinary lift in certainty through a feeling of achievement. You ought to likewise attempt and accomplish something you're great at any rate once every day. Regardless of whether you're a specialist at playing an instrument or you have a remarkable ability for a computer game, take a break from your calendar and do it. It'll be an incredible assistance.

Another life-changing change you can make is to counterfeit it. This may sound hard, yet this works extraordinary. Imagine that you're a character you know, who is smart, intelligent, and sure about themselves. Maybe you know one from a TV program, a motion picture or a book. Feel free to convey all that you state with certainty, regardless of whether you don't know of it, or you're panicked. You'll see that as you counterfeit it to an ever-increasing extent, in the end, you acquire that trust, in actuality.

## Give up

Endeavoring to control every one of incredible results is, without a doubt, the fundamental driver for compensation. Since when you do, you are likewise destined to hotly consider what to do in each snapshot of your life in dread of what could like this occur straightaway. The best thing you can do is to persuade yourself not to. Understand that you have nothing to do with what happens in your life, and thus, there is no motivation to stress over it. The universe has your destiny chosen, so you should make the most out of each minute. Attempt and understand this before anything you may falter do, and it'll assist you with stopping overthinking and take care of business.

Something else you can do make explicit time allotments to settle on any choice. Regardless of whether it is to proceed to converse with somebody or more significant life decisions which may constrain you to overthink. Pause for a moment for the little ones and a couple of days for the bigger ones in life and no more. This would push you to survey a choice usually and research to settle on the ideal decision. When you do decide on an opportunity, steel yourself and do what needs to be done. It may scare yet you'll see it remunerating toward the end.

By the day's end, the most significant piece to acknowledge is that we as a whole hold the possibility to accomplish all that we have longed for, and the main thing we need to do is to steel ourselves and evacuate our hindrances. What's more, that has a significant effect.

# Quit Overthinking and Causing Yourself Anxiety - Here's How to Make Things More Manageable

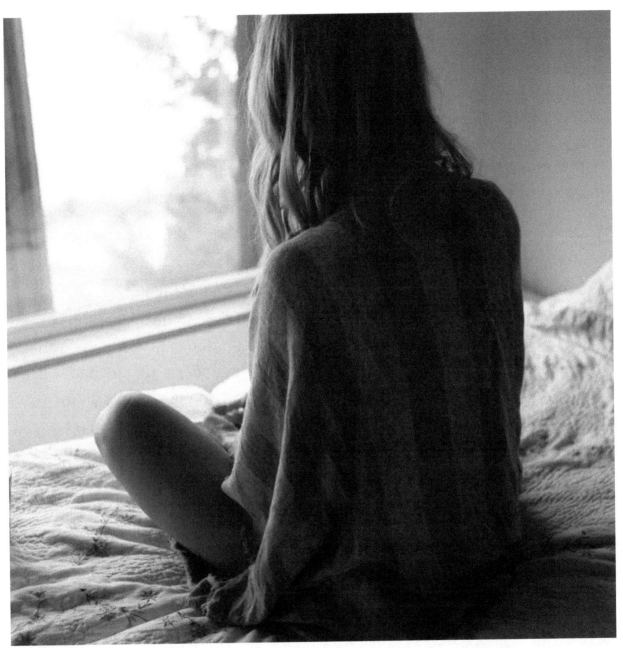

Separate it. The ideal approach to quit overthinking is to break enormous targets or objectives into littler assignments. Put the errands that are basic to your goal higher up on the need list. Along these lines, you'll begin doing the most significant and squeezing things to get your objective finished. When you start finding what's most significant in reaching your goal finished, you've done a large portion of the work, and you'll begin to turn out to be less on edge about completing the work.

Try not to overpower yourself. This can cause significantly more tension. It is effortless for us to perceive how hard an assignment will be to finished. It's human instinct to be overpowered. When you place yourself in this circumstance, you're just making lethality towards finishing the activity. Negative considerations or potentially activities can make you backtrack on what you're endeavoring to do. Stop yourself in case you're getting in the propensity for changing each seemingly insignificant detail that has to do

with completing the job needing to be done. As referenced above, do the most significant things first and proceed onward once finished.


Agent undertakings. There are a few things that are impossible alone. Now and then, you don't have room schedule-wise or the ability essential to complete a task. That is alright. This is the ideal time to designate those undertakings to somebody who has the time or aptitudes to complete it for you. This is particularly significant in case you're under a set due date. There's nothing superior to having another person do the snort work for you while you deal with the more significant strides to completing the current task. Doing this will likewise enable you to decrease pressure; along these lines, you become less on edge.

# Managing Life and Over-Thinking

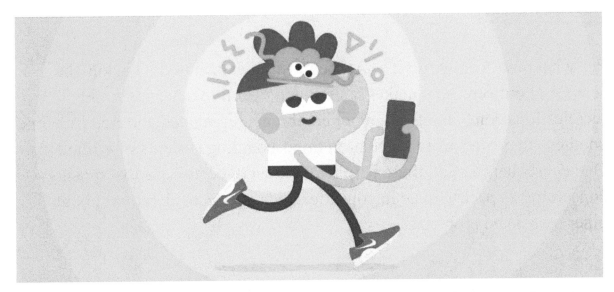

After all the diligent work, this ought to be the season when we at long last quit worrying and begin having fun. How would you stop those annoying 'imagine a scenario where?' stresses are swarming back.

We as a whole do it once in a while - stress over things we've said or done, examine disposable remarks others have or invest hours dismembering the significance of a specific email or letter. Nearly without acknowledging it, we get sucked into a winding of negative contemplations and feelings that take our delight and excitement. It's an example that a few clinicians bring over reasoning. The underlying considerations lead to progressively negative musings, the inquiries to more inquiries. The over reasoning turns into a course that matures and fabricates so that everything gains out of power. Stall out in this negative cycle, and it can influence your life. It can likewise prompt some downright awful choices when generally little issues turn out to be so dramatically overemphasized that you lose your point of view on them.

When we over think-focusing on what has occurred previously (future) - we are obliterating the minute we are in. You pass up encountering and appreciating the present time and place of your life.

For what reason do we do it? - At the most fundamental dimension, the science of our cerebrum makes it simple to over think. Musings and recollections don't merely sit in our cerebrums segregated and free from one another - they are woven together in mind-boggling systems of affiliations. One consequence of all these perplexing interconnections is that musings concerning a specific issue in your life can trigger considerations about other associated problems.

A large portion of us have some negative recollections, stresses over the future, or worries about the present. A significant part of the time we're most likely not aware of these negative musings. In any case, when they come over us, regardless of whether it's because the climate's terrible or because we alcoholic an excessive amount of wine, it's simpler to review the negative recollections and start the cycle of over reasoning. Numerous ladies are over-burden with juggling home and work responsibilities and want to do everything superbly. We will, in general feel in charge of everybody, a figure we ought to be in charge and set ourselves strangely particular requirements.

How to defeat it? - If you're endless over scholar, just being advised to invest significant time and unwind won't do it for you. You have to find a way to control and conquer contrary reasoning. Ending the propensity isn't simple, and there's no enchantment answer for everybody, except these are a portion of the means that specialists propose can enable you to break out of the negative cycle of over reasoning.

**1. Offer yourself a reprieve -** Free your brain with something that draws in your fixation and lifts your mindset - regardless of whether it's perusing a decent book, strolling the canine, having a back rub or doing the rec center.

**2. Take yourself close by -** When you see yourself going over similar musings, let yourself know immovably to stop — post yellow stickers around your work area and the house as updates.

**3. Jettison the postponing strategies -** If there are specific circumstances or spots that trigger over reasoning, for example, a work area heaped high with papers or open letters or messages, at that point take care of business, anyway little. Over reasoning that is connected with inertia can turn into an endless loop. Rather than living in dread of what you can't do and what could occur, it's far superior to handle it virtually by accomplishing something.

**4. Discharge your contemplations -** Issues that expect large extents after frantic stressing can all of a sudden dissolve away when you talk them through with a companion. They can appear to be absurd or even amusing. Making a joke out of them can genuinely defuse your stresses.

**5. Plan for deduction time -** choose when you enable yourself to think. Point of confinement the time you give yourself and adhere to your timetable. Envision keeping every one of those contemplations in a single box that you can take out at a specific time, at that point seal and put it away when the time runs out.

**6. Appreciate the occasion -** Actively plan things that you understand. It doesn't make a difference what it is - whatever works for you. It's difficult to grieve in negative over reasoning when you're having some good times.

**7. Express your feelings** - Instead of going into a profound examination of what your feelings truly mean, enable yourself to encounter them for a change. Sob, shout, punch a pad, will allow yourself to feel the warmth and after that proceed onward.

**8. Pardon yourself** - That doesn't mean imagining that slight or harmful comments never occurred, yet it means settling on a decision to set them aside as opposed to harp on them.

**9. Be careful** - Take time every day to be at the time. It won't be simple, however, persevere, and you'll receive the benefits. Go out in the greenhouse to watch the dusk, go through 15 minutes in the recreation center at noon or sit in a bistro all alone. Try not to exile the considerations, let them travel every which way, yet see what's near and how your body feels.

# Positive Attitude Tips - 3 Fast & Effective Tips to Change Negative Thinking

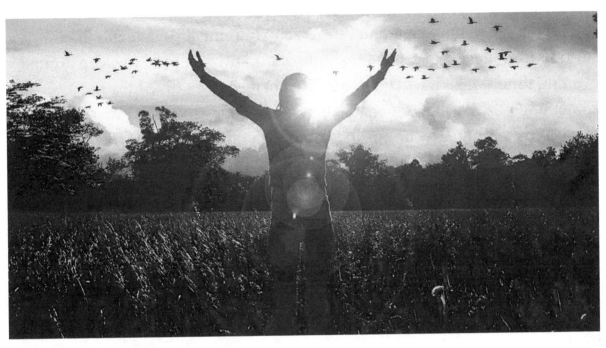

**Uplifting Attitude Tips:**

Do you ever consider how or why you get so cynical about existence all in all? Well, that isn't elusive the response to this inquiry. It is genuinely situated to a limited extent on how you invest your energy and who you invest your time with. For example, when you spend your energy in adverse situations and around negative individuals, at that point, you will, in all probability, end up with a lot of negative musings.

If you are somebody that is having issues and continually battling a negative frame of mind and need to think increasingly positive at that point, read this whole section on uplifting mentality tips. They have helped many individuals, and they can genuinely support you if you begin to apply them in your day by day life.

# Here are 3 Fast and Effective Tips to Change Negative Thinking.

1. Truly begin to make it a point to screen your musings and emotions starting from the exact second that you get up till you head to sleep around evening time. Make it a need to quickly change a negative idea to something positive and not enable that negative idea to wait. You can do this by concentrating your musings on what you need as opposed to focus on what you don't need throughout everyday life.

2. Remain in the organization of playful constructive individuals and indeed point of confinement or control back your time with other people who are always negative about everything. This is hugely significant because that is a large piece of how you end up having a negative frame of mind in any case.

3. Make a rundown of at any rate three things that you are appreciative for throughout everyday life. This can be your wellbeing, your activity or profession, or the way that you have a rooftop over your head. At that point, when you feel depressed, to consider the things that you must be appreciative for and center around them rather than the negative considerations that you were having.

**Step by step instructions to Change Negative Thinking: 3 Tips to Develop A Positive Attitude**

Figuring out how to change contrary reasoning into constructive contemplations isn't as simple as it sounds, particularly for specific individuals who have been so used to harping on the discouraging and frustrating pieces of life.

While the facts confirm that we make our very own world and that we pick how we see it, now and again we can't prevent ourselves from concentrating on the terrible things.

If you are baffled, disappointed, and need to know how to change contrary reasoning, here are a couple of tips that could help.

## Tip # 1: Don't Generalize.

Not all things are bound to turn out badly when one awful thing occurs. Overstating the situation can aggravate you feel and make you stress over things you shouldn't be.

Acknowledge the way that you can't control everything, and not all things can go how you need them to. Pick, instead, to locate the positive in each situation.

Concentrate on the things that you can change. Keeping a receptive outlook will help you in figuring out how to change contrary reasoning.

## Tip # 2: Don't Jump into Conclusions.

Right when looked with a problematic situation, make a stride back, and discover what the remainder of the story is. Taking a gander at conditions in a comprehensive and segregated way will enable you to get all the fundamental data on the issue, with the goal that you can be increasingly arranged to approach and explain it.

Going overboard on little subtleties won't help and will make you feel troubled. Once more, keeping an open point of view will place you in a superior position to respond and react suitably.

**Tip # 3: Don't Take Everything Personally.**

Figure out how to change contrary reasoning by realizing how to separate what is coordinated towards you as an individual, from that which is organized towards the situation.

In all honesty, not all things are about you. Try not to let dread, neurosis, or weakness assume control over you and cause you to trust that each negative remark or activity is coordinated towards you.

Contributing an excessive amount of feeling (on issues that don't require it) will cause you to lose center around the more significant things. Instead, direct your consideration and spend your vitality on improving what you can in the situation.

The most significant thing in figuring out how to change contrary reasoning is to recollect that beneficial things do occur in spite of difficulties, frustrations, disappointments, and torment. As the expression goes, you can concentrate on what's going on in your life, or you can focus on what's the right side.

# The most effective method to Change Negative Thinking into Positive Thinking with Self-Talk

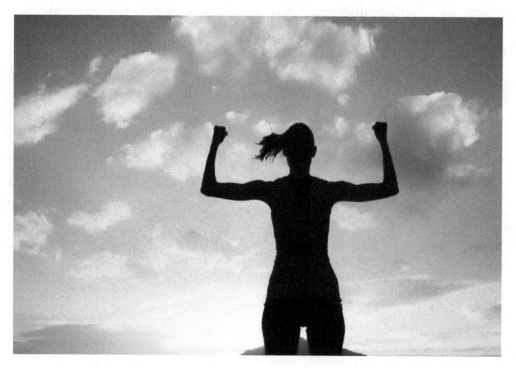

Have you at any experienced point occasions where a perpetual progression of humming jabber bothers at you in your brain? If it was another person, it is futile to attempt and get it. However, you can. You comprehend what that spout of musings is stating because everything originates from inside you.

That voice in your mind, the inward judge, when you either war or mull over with yourself is self-talk. You it is possible that you gave it a chance to annoy away and cut you down, or you can utilize it to psych yourself up and let it help you face life's difficulties head-on. What is the mystery? What is power? How would you figure out how to change contrary reasoning into positive reasoning?

# The Power

It might be a "duh" commendable proclamation however we do neglect to understand that the kinds of considerations we think pretty much go about as an antecedent of what state of mind we'll be in. If you believe tragic or distraught musings, at that point you feel such. When you feel upbeat, it isn't challenging to be. This is simply the thought behind the idea of an inevitable outcome. Think you'll fizzle, and you most likely will as you feel moving in the direction of your objective as inconsequential. If you think you succeed, your odds of doing as such go up.

# Spotting Destruction

With figuring out how to change contrary reasoning into positive reasoning, you should comprehend what it is you do with your musings that aren't so useful. There are numerous types of negative self-talk, one of which is a great one - envisioning the more terrible. Although there is a platitude which instructs us to "get ready for the most noticeably terrible and trust in the best," ensure you satisfy the two pieces of the arrangement and not favor one side — another future seeing things in absolutes. You're either fruitful or a thundering disappointment, positive or negative with no dark areas. Accusing yourself is additionally a terrible reasoning propensity. At last, there's where you channel everything and center around the negative and dismissal the positive. Attempt your best to veer far from these kinds of considerations

## The Change Tips

Furthermore, presently, we have the headliner - how to change contrary reasoning into positive reasoning. This is a genuinely essential undertaking; you must be focused on following this training and make a propensity out of it. To begin with, stop to investigate exactly what you're making of. Attempt to see the positive qualities in things or even test yourself too. Following that, why not see the humor in something every day in spite of the harsh occasions. This would leave you feeling less pushed. Last, carry on with a decent life in body, organization, and psyche. Eat well and exercise too, encircle yourself with constructive individuals and let it rub on you, and practice positive self-talk.

Changing from negative to positive reasoning doesn't occur without any forethought. It takes practice. Never lose expectation or heart. Take this test and gain from it well.

# CHAPTER TWO

## Stop Negative Thinking in Its Tracks - 3 Simple Stress Management Tips for a Positive Attitude

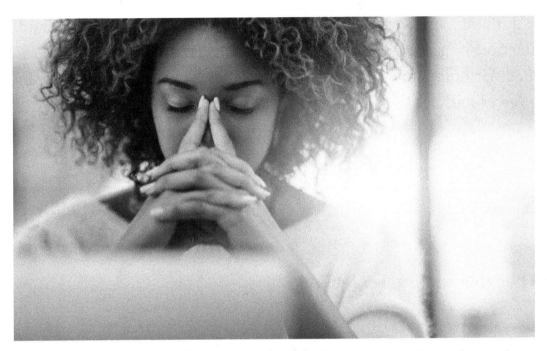

Most business people and solopreneurs that I encourage experience issues with regards to having the option to stop adverse reasoning. Negative thoughts can cost you a group in accomplishing your objective of monetary achievement.

Negative frames of mind and thoughts discharge a toxic substance into our bodies, and that causes greater antagonism and sentiments of grief. This prepares for disappointment, dissatisfactions, and dissatisfactions.

There are a few minimal known assets, tips thoughts that not exclusively can spare you a considerable amount of cash; however, make your dream reasonable. Also, I am going to uncover three straightforward pressure the board tips to stop contrary reasoning.

## #1: Smile

If you have been brought up in toxic air, it might be troublesome at first to begin thinking positively. The initial step is to grin more. A grin is said to be infectious. Take a stab at smiling at an outsider and check whether it is returned. Grinning gives you a more beneficial feeling of prosperity, and it takes fewer muscles than scowling!

## #2: Thoughts and frame of mind

Thoughts and frames of mind can't be changed in a moment or even overnight. It takes work to make your account mindful that it is thoroughly considering negative thoughts or putting negative pictures.

It must be prepared to think just significant and positive thoughts — picture positive results to the circumstances throughout your life.

This will take tolerance and determination, and it is something that should be dealt with consistently. Before long, positive reasoning will turn out to be progressively characteristic, and you will think great thoughts automatically.

## #3: Visualization

Perception is an excellent method for transforming negative thoughts into positive ones.

At the point when a circumstance springs up, take a gander at it and enable your brain to see a positive result. Anticipate that things should work out as opposed to imagining the most exceedingly awful possible outcome.

You may trust the intensity of positive reasoning is a fantasy or a legend. Why out it a go after only a couple of days or seven days.

Check whether your mentality will change toward your conditions.

Keep in mind, definite draws in positive.

Grin often! It might transform you and help you accomplish your fantasies.

One of the most significant impediments that anticipate business people and solopreneurs from having the option to quit thinking pessimistic is that they are excessively occupied.

**Inspirational Attitude Tips - 5 Easy Steps to Stop Negative Thinking**

We live in such a cynical world read the newspapers and watch the news on TV. This does not successfully rouse or elevate us in a positive manner. What you center around in life decides your attitude, and on the off chance that those negative thoughts attack your psyche, at that point you will turn out to be exceptionally despondent.

If you are somebody having issues beating a negative disposition, at that point, read this article and apply the basic uplifting frame of mind tips in your day by day life. They have genuinely helped many individuals have a progressively uplifting frame of mind and a more joyful life.

**Here are 5 Easy Steps to Stop Negative Thinking.**

1. Peruse and tune in to positive learning material regularly as opposed to perusing or tuning in to the news in newspapers or on the TV. This will truly change your progressively positive demeanor.

2. Avoid pessimistic people, whether this is your family, companion, or colleague. You cannot bear to become involved with their pessimism. Since it will just bring you down in your own life, only enable yourself to keep organization with people with an uplifting frame of mind.

3. Maintain a strategic distance from negative situations they unequivocally impact your state of mind and how you are feeling. On the off chance that you pick favorable conditions that are elevating and moving, at that point, you will, in general, have an increasingly uplifting mentality.

4. Abstain from concentrating on negative things in your regular day to day existence. Concentrate on what you need in life, not on what you don't need throughout everyday life.

5. Abstain from investing your energy in exercises that don't concur with what you need throughout everyday life. In such a case that you get all made up for the lost time in things that are not imperative to you. At that

point, you will be vexed that you didn't accomplish the things that are increasingly essential to you. The significant thing is to reliably be taking a shot at or towards the exercises that will make your life what you need, and this thus will enable you to have an uplifting disposition.

When you are not content with your life, at that point, it is dependent upon you to transform it.

# Defeating Negative Thinking - 6 Tips on How to Be a Positive Person

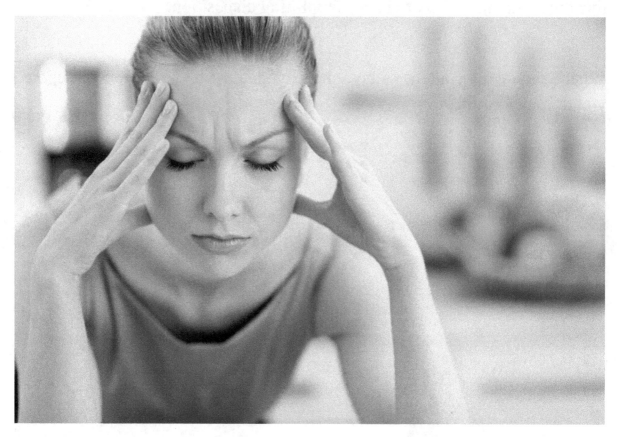

A constructive individual is one that numerous people would need to be with, and many would need to be around with. A significant number of us need to get that positive emanation that causes us to feel better and encourages us to see lovely and positive things throughout everyday life.

There is a lot of contrary occasions and things occurring on the planet now and taking a gander at it in a pessimistic individual's eyes can make life all the more discouraging and disappointing, and without a doubt, you don't need that to transpire.

If you are endeavoring to take out negative thoughts in your psyche and you are searching for courses in beating contrary reasoning, here are a couple of tips that you may discover valuable.

1. Have command over your feelings. A flood of passion often placed you into a circumstance where you can't control yourself, and you may finish up doing negative things that you would most likely lament later. Life has for sure a lot of difficulties and disagreeable astonishments, and once you experience one, you will no doubt be unfit to control your emotions and marginally put yourself into a cheerful misstep of negative assessments. If you can deal with your feelings, you can likewise help yourself in beating these negatives throughout everyday life and become a superior, increasingly constructive individual.

2. Discover approaches to help other people every day, even in your very own little ways. Another tip that can help you in defeating contrary reasoning is to discover time to help other people. By giving and helping, you can support yourself create positive propensities, and obviously, it will likewise give you an increase in positive vitality. Giving and helping other people will likewise enable you to understand that your issues are excessively little contrasted with what others are also having.

3. Be aware of utilizing positive words rather than those negative ones. You may not know it, but instead, there are a ton of essential negative words used every day, and they can get negative impacts to your attitude also. The more you state that your life is distressing or you are, or you are unfortunate enough, the more that these things will transpire.

4. Figure out how to tune in to positive melodies, positive stories and figure out how to maintain a strategic distance from tattle no matter what. Indeed,

the things you hear, see and look about you are incredible impacts in your attitude and when are always tuning in to negative and discouraging melodies and tattles, the more you will likewise be affected by them.

5. **Make it a standard to not gripe or whimper.** Grumbling or crying might be unavoidable in this life mainly if things don't go your specific manner yet on the off chance that you continued griping and whimpering, you can likewise develop this unfortunate propensity and will lead you to turn into an antagonistic individual who dependably observes something negative out of something.

6. **Go with constructive people.** Indeed, one of the least demanding approaches to be a productive individual is to be encompassed by helpful people and be related to them. Uplifting mentality and an inspirational standpoint are often infectious. If you oblige constructive people, you will likewise be one of them, along these lines try to recognize what kinds of people you are going out with.

These are only 6 of the things that you can remember whether you need to beat contrary reasoning. Likewise, remember that you can to be sure conquered negative idea designs and appreciate a more joyful life.

# Positive Attitude Tips - 5 Simple Steps to Overcome Negative Thinking

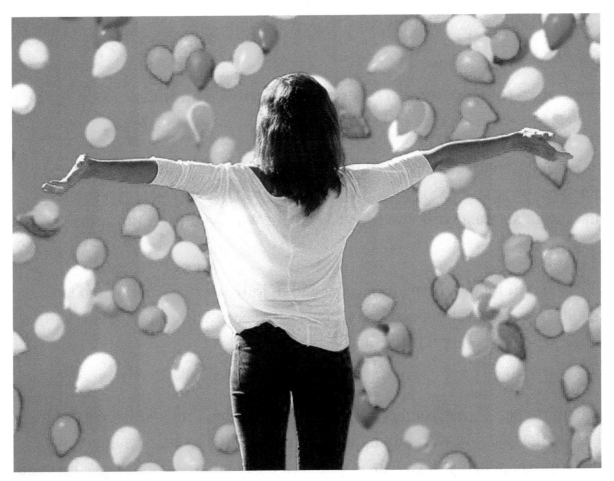

These positive demeanor tips will roll out an improvement in your life and help you to conquer contrary reasoning, which is the thing that keeps you down throughout everyday life. The funny thing in the public eye is the way that individuals are so troubled in their life. That is, for the most part since they are so overwhelmed with contrary reasoning that they cannot perceive what is feasible for themselves. If they would figure out how to apply the significant strides to defeat contrary thinking, then their lives would be loaded with joy and achievement.

If you are somebody, who is continually attempting to beat contrary reasoning, at that point set aside the effort to get familiar with the essential positive demeanor tips in this section, when you do and, at that point, proceed to apply them, you will before long observe a positive change in your life and know precisely how to defeat contrary reasoning.

**Here are 5 Simple Steps to Overcome Negative Thinking.**

1. Try not to harp on negative things. Instead, think about something positive for yourself. Since you become a result of what you invest energy making of so make your idea positive about what you need for yourself.

2. Try not to invest energy around negative individuals. Since you become a result of the general population, you invest energy with so associate with other people who are positive and playful.

3. Comprehend what you need throughout everyday life and have a course. This will assist you with having something positive to take a stab at and accomplish. When you psyche is centered on great positive things, then you will see that you won't have negative musings.

4. Set objectives for yourself all the time for all parts of your life. This keeps you centered throughout everyday life and keeps you on track to accomplishing what you truly need.

5. Keep your regions that you invest a ton of energy in spotless and flawless and efficient so when you need something you can without much of a stretch discover it. Again, you become a result of your condition, so if you

are in a positive, clean, efficient zone, it will have a positive effect in your life. I trust these positive demeanor tips are useful to you.

# Intellectual Therapy - Top 7 Tips to Untwist Your Thinking

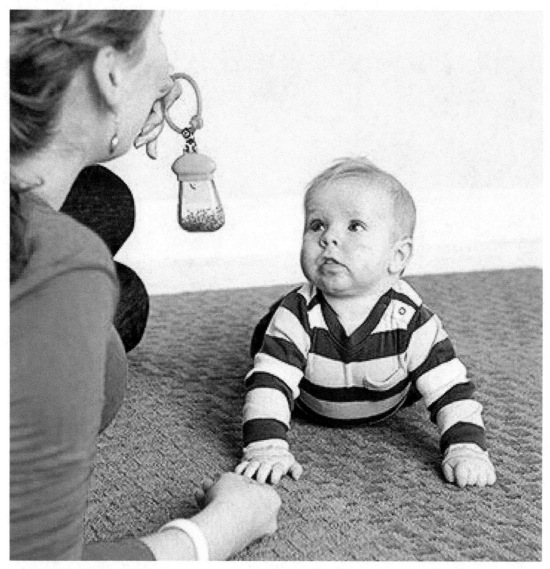

When you feel awful, your reasoning winds up negative. This is the ABC of feeling. 'A' represents the Actual occasion, 'B' for your Beliefs about it and 'C' for the Consequences you experience on account of their convictions. When you can find some way, or another keep false negative confidences from conforming to a specific occasion, you have gone far toward securing yourself structure the pointless negative feelings that are certain to pursue from such misshaped thinking. I prescribe seven hints to shield yourself from negative, contorted reasoning. These tips work for some unpleasant encounters, yet how about we use, for instance, especially unpleasant encounters, yet how about we use, for example, an especially nasty separation. In the throes of a frightful divorce, you may be enticed to trust vast numbers of the charges your ex levels against you: You're childish, cutthroat and sinister, and not just that, you are lousy in bed. If you become tied up with this image of yourself, the results likely could be low confidence and blame, also severe dejection. Psychological treatment attempts to change the Bs - your convictions - so you don't encounter the Cs - negative results. Here's how to adapt.

## 1. Characterize Your Terms

You had no thoughts your ex had illicit relationships. You were visually impaired. Characterize daze. The word reference says, "totally without sight." That wasn't you. You saw that your ex was pulled back from you and was investing a considerable measure of energy "working late." You weren't visually impaired, just excessively trusting of somebody you had each motivation to accept reliable.

## 2. Take care of The Problem

You exploded when you got back home early and found your ex, who moved out months prior, out of the blue in your home. Since that revolting scene, you have felt that your "awful temper" has transformed you into a "beast." Possibly, however, the issue for this situation isn't your temper. The genuine issue is that your ex still has keys to your home. Perhaps the time has come to change the locks.

### 3. Take A Survey

Your ex demands that your refusal to take the children for an additional day following an occasion end of the week demonstrates you are malicious. You keep up that you are available to a rescheduling time with the kids, yet not when the genuine reason is to enable your ex to stream off to a lavish retreat with another sweetheart. You feel defended, however after a shouting contention on the telephone, and your certainty is shaken. Maybe you are a malicious wet blanket. Presently an ideal opportunity to call a couple of companions and request their perspectives. Odds are they will say you are legitimized.

### 4. Converse with Yourself as You Would to A Best Friend

Assume a companion was getting separated and felt like an egotistical, cruel, evil disappointment. What might you say? Most likely, something like You is not a disappointment just because your relationship finished. Many relational unions end in separation, and many winning groups lose a game every so often. It is harsh to bear a divorce, and separations failing to bring out the best in individuals, yet I have known you for a considerable length of time, and you are a warm, kind, mindful individual.

### 5. Look at The Evidence

Take in the 10,000-foot view. Record it if you need to. Your ex says you are lousy in bed; however, would you say you are true? Until you learned of your ex's unfaithfulness, you two had an excellent sexual relationship. After your heart was broken, you didn't have any vitality for sex, particularly with the individual who rejected you. That isn't being lousy in bed. That is a typical response to selling out.

## 6. Search for Partial Successes

Rather than believing that your marriage was a finished disappointment, consider the numerous ways that it was effective: You alternated putting each other through school, and now you both have substantially more satisfying professions than you had when you met. You have two incredible children, and the issues that prompted your separation have given you essential new bits of knowledge into the sort of individual you will search for in your next relationship.

## 7. Test

Perceive how this contrary reasoning about yourself in this one region piles facing your conduct in different territories. Your ex called you childish for needing to keep the house, however, would you say you are true? When you were narrow-minded, you wouldn't provide for philanthropy, wouldn't help companions out of luck and wouldn't share credit for your gathering's achievements at work. Test your responses whenever a beneficent requesting arrives, or a companion calls with an issue or your collective endeavors are perceived. When you compose a check, offer to help out or acclaim an associate, you are not by any means childish. You may not be as unselfish as you prefer to be. However, you are not the monstrosity your ex says you are.

# How to Avoid Negative Thinking

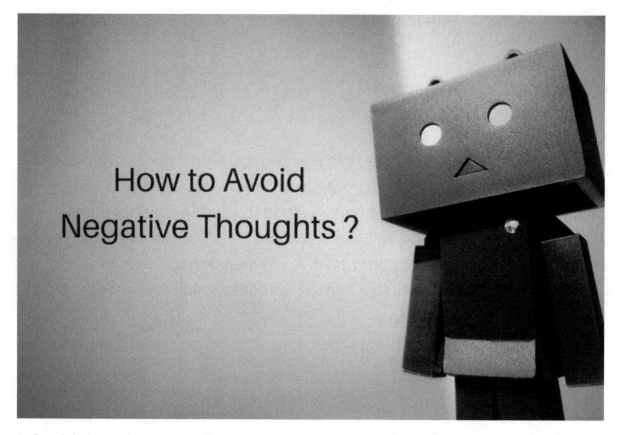

It is alright to be stressed over something. Nobody truly holds the future, isn't that so? You ought to be frightened, however, if your stress is assuming control over your whole existence. You can never again work so well. You don't seek after specific exercises since you are excessively terrified of fizzling.

Is there an approach to escape this contrary reasoning? Honestly, there is. You can attempt these thoughts:

1. Gain from the legends. Do you realize that there are a large number of individuals who bombed before they succeeded? Take Abraham Lincoln, for instance. Before he conveyed the famous Gettysburg, Address and

turned into a hero for majority rules system, he had a few political mishaps. He lost a lot of races.

A few entertainers needed to maintain odd sources of income before they set up themselves in Hollywood. Sandra Bullock filled in as a server, and coat checks young lady, and barkeep before she was given her Best Actress Award. When these individuals enable contrary reasoning to command them, they won't make extraordinary progress in their lives. You ought to do the equivalent as well.

2. Get yourself occupied. You offer yourself a chance to engage negative thoughts if you are inert. There is nothing else a lot to do. To maintain a strategic distance from that, participate in a few exercises. Seek after the same number of things as you like. You can go to class, play sports, head on to an exercise center, get together with companions, and enable your innovative procedure to allow you to get by.

3. Use assertions. You can likewise utilize subliminal messages to enable you to get by. Observe the accompanying articulations:

- I can improve my dimension of self-assurance.
- I don't need to stress over tomorrow.
- I anticipate a fresh start each day.
- I let go of the past and grasp the present.
- I abide right now.

What do you see about these announcements? The more that you discuss these subliminal messages, the more they become realities to you. These subliminal messages can change your way of reasoning. You will be progressively open to new thoughts and, the majority of all, remain in the present, where you don't need to consider what's to come.

4. Begin tolerating reality. In all actuality, you don't generally have much power about what's to come. You can put forth a valiant effort. It is just when you can begin tolerating the reality you have no full control over what will happen you start to live more joyfully. Appreciate the existence you at present have at this moment.

5. Burrow further on the reason for your stress. For what reason would you say you are so stressed? Is it true that you are frightened you will get an intense sickness? At that point, deal with yourself more. Do you believe you want toward the end in your present employment? Investigate better chances and take up intriguing classes to sharpen your aptitudes.

Negative thoughts can worry you, making you feel worn out, discouraged, and dismal a lot of times. Much as could sensibly be healthy, you ought to figure out how to conquer them by observing the previously mentioned tips.

**Four Tips to Confront Negative Mindsets**

**1. Don't overthink**

There is nothing more burdensome and harmful than overthinking. When you overthink, your cerebrum is too jumbled even to consider is taking care of business. Your inspirations vary, and before the day's over, you may, in any case, be uncertain what your needs are. This is exceptionally regular of this sort of mentality.

A standout amongst the ideal ways not to overthink is to set aside some effort to ponder. Indeed, even 20 minutes of contemplation daily will hinder your negative reasoning examples and help you center around what is generally significant. Attempt it for half a month and notice the adjustment in your overthinking designs.

## 2. See openings, not issues

Scholars are an exceptionally touchy gathering of people. We will, in general, frequently be very harmful, and we center around the issues and feel caught by them. Also, this can set us in the mood for seeing and translating everything negatively. Despite what things transpire each day, from dismissals to only not having the option to finish our day by day word tallies, we decipher these things in negative terms.

Nonetheless, when we change our reasoning examples from negative to progressively idealistic ones and see each issue as an open door for learning, our psychological exhibition improves, and we will, in general, be significantly increasingly satisfied and profitable. There are exercises embedded in every one of our issues. We should set aside the effort to figure out what they are.

## 3. Envision Doing What Seems Impossible

The most significant thing that journalists can accomplish for themselves is to envision that they will achieve something that causes them incredible dread, for example, sending original copies out to distributors. That way, an essayist can feel increasingly positive about conveying her composition, and she can envision how great she will feel after she has sent the original copy.

## 4. Stand up to negative thoughts head on

Here and there we can be the cause of all our problems. We can concentrate on the entirety of our negative thoughts about what we're not doing right. This can make examples of contrary reasoning that can keep going quite a while in case we're not cautious. In this manner, it is essential for scholars to stop negative thoughts in their tracks. Remember, you're only another bloom, and you're attempting to adapt to a troublesome situation. You can do it, yet it will be tough to do as such at first.

By following these tips, you will find a way to keep away from negative thoughts and mentalities. This will improve your inventiveness and generally speaking profitability. Also, this is a success win for all authors.

We, as a whole need to be glad and substance scholars. We can be by finding a way to be individual and confident authors, one minute on end.

# CHAPTER THREE
## Negative Thinking Disorders

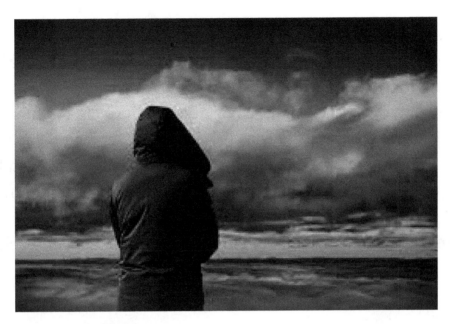

**It's Not Beware; It's Be Aware**

Contrary reasoning issue is disarranged that branch from extreme nervousness and is most usually named as tension issue. Under this specific sort of turmoil are disarranges like over the top urgent issue, summed up tension issue, post-horrendous pressure, alarm issue, and social fear. It's the contrary reasoning in these negative reasoning issue or nervousness issue that feeds the uneasiness making it develop. This issue is established in our considerations. To fix it, we should change our negative musings into positive ones with ways like subjective treatment.

**It's All the Same and Holding On**

People who experience the evil impacts of such contrary reasoning issue trust that everything will remain the equivalent and it would dependably be awful - nothing changes. By taking such a conviction into their arrangement of reasoning, they're shutting entryways or approaches to get help. Treatment for such issue is a usual procedure and by clutching their point.

Discussing hanging tight, with these sorts of disarranges, individuals experiencing it clutch damaging or horrendous encounters. Like this, they make it harder for themselves to get away from the endless loop of antagonism and nervousness. These negative musings are the fundamental power wellspring of these scatters as they are never-ending being an idea of. It's one thing to clutch a memory, yet another circumstance totally when you fixate on it and fall caught to a destructive idea cycle. In addition to the fact that it interrupts your everyday life, it additionally alters your rationale and may make you avoid certain circumstances and in actuality constrain you.

## Absolutes

Those experiencing contrary reasoning issue think in absolutes or limits. They see that there must be a terrible or decent circumstance. This can be especially hard to manage as they, as a rule, see the negative piece of things more and amplify them, eclipsing whatever positive there is. To change by the typical idea, they should comprehend that stressing is typical to a degree and that there would dependably be upsides and downsides or tremendous and awful in the circumstances. They should realize that whatever con or terrible there is ought not to control or restrict them. They should discover what it is that is causing them the fits of anxiety and fanatical reasoning and abstain from inclination defenseless or powerless. We should all understand that we are in charge.

Contrary reasoning issue may take various structures and extents, yet one component remains the equivalent - the contrary reasoning. The drug may help; however, by the day's end, whatever occurs, it's something we need to deal with in our brains. Early mediation is ideal and is available to treatment would ensure that advancement would move along as it should. Life is great, it may not be simple, but instead, it is excellent. Find it.

**Habitual Thinking Disorder**

**Battle It!**

It happens over and over and once more. Your contemplations appear to spin around very similar things over and over. It's expending you gradually. You endeavor to rest. However, you can't. There's a humming, a pestering, an irritating voice in your mind that won't give you harmony. It frequents you. You can't complete anything. You realize it needs to stop. This, old buddy, is the indication of the formal reasoning issue.

**I'll Never Get over It.**

Getting over the impulsive reasoning issue is an assignment with the trouble that is equal to its seriousness. A couple of troubling musings are satisfactory and particularly typical. Having considerations that appear to assume control over your life; however, giving it a chance to leave you speechless as opposed to moving relentlessly forward is very unfortunate. It's downright awful when you let it drag you to the past and keep you there.

All things being equal, it is anything but difficult to overcome this issue. You truly need to need it, and you should be eager to focus on beating it because there's a straightforward arrangement that can posture to be extremely troublesome if you go on about it with the methods for an enthusiastic reasoning issue. What's going on here? It's merely to concentrate on positive contemplations and have faith in them. Make a decent attempt to bring yourself harmony. Once more, everything's more complicated than one might expect, particularly with a positive frame of mind conceived from this issue.

**Goodness Yeah? So, what's the Plan?**

The best arrangement you could need to overcome mechanical reasoning issue is to endeavor to slaughter each negative idea when it comes. When you see that your musings are beginning to get sharp, go for a positive reply. You can believe, "I'm not going to have a ton of fun at the gathering" at that point go "however, on the other hand, my companions are there so it'll be alright. It very well may be more than alright." It might be challenging to do at first from its sheer newness, and how it's so inverse to what you're utilized to, yet like-minded all abilities, all you need is a touch of training. Help yourself out and don't lose heart with this one. The more you do it, the more straightforward it gets and the more it'd appear to be a programmed reflex.

Beating critical reasoning issue is your opportunity not merely to better your state of mind or yourself as an individual, yet it can better your life when all is said in done. Before long you'd discover things looking into your way and that you're getting to places you need to be throughout everyday life. Escape the shadows; see life in a different light.

**Positive or Negative Thinking**

As of now, you can discover sufficient proof to demonstrate that your life is hopeless, exhausting, and discouraging. You can likewise create evidence to prove that your life is happy and energizing.

**We should complete an activity!**

Check out the room you are in. Do you see any residue and soil? Any turmoil? A storage room or drawers that need arranging? A heap of papers that ought to be recorded or reused? Does the room need paint or fix? Is the light switch plate smeared?

How would you feel? Did you discover enough proof that life is dreadful, discouraging, and an excessive amount to deal with?

Check out the room once more. Do you see something given by a companion or relative that is exceptional to you? Does it bring sweet recollections? If you are perched on an agreeable seat? Do you have a PC to keep in contact with companions and become familiar with a wide range of energizing things? Do you have flooring that is more pleasant than an earth floor? Anything there that produces music for you? Compact disc player, radio? It isn't great that we can flip that switch and have light whenever of day or night?

How would you feel now? Did you discover enough proof that life is fantastic, brilliant, and brimming with beneficial things?

Our musings are powerful! Those musings control hormones in our body, and those hormones make us feel better or awful. They additionally decide if we have great wellbeing or horrendous wellbeing, regardless of whether we are discouraged or euphoric.

Indeed, there is a concoction irregularity when individuals are discouraged, yet we should inquire as to why? God did not make us that way. There is lot of research out there on what considerations to do our wellbeing.

If you checked out the room and didn't discover anything significant that didn't come without a miserable or negative idea, I would state that you don't feel sound in that condition of reasoning. It takes a noteworthy upgrade to get your "stinking reasoning" out the entryway, yet you can do it!

Shouldn't something be said about positive reasoning? That can be similarly as awful for you!

Positive scholars now and again utilize positive reasoning as an approach to legitimize their failure to acknowledge the occasion. They have a considerable rundown of "should," and except if their conditions coordinate with flawlessness (and it once in a while does), they retreat into positive musings, supposing they will give a superior world to everybody with positive articulations.

Some positive masterminds have a heavenly sounding type of forswearing.

"To concentrate on the positive isn't to slight certain notice sign of a "negative" sort that, whenever disregarded, in the end, lead to burden, best case scenario, and catastrophe even from a pessimistic standpoint. When we utilize these negative signs to maintain a strategic distance from calamity, at that point, they're not negative all things considered. "

On account of illness, we can recognize the indications of sickness and get familiar with everything we can to defeat that ailment and move towards that objective. Or then again, we can start by saying that "we have" that infection. In the wake of asserting it as our own long enough, our mind will in general trust it, and our body might be less inclined to dispose of it.

We are advised to live at the time. However, a large portion of us is thinking about the past and additionally the future a large part of the day, so when we will do this, at any rate, make it beautiful. Think about the beneficial things from an earlier time and the useful things that will occur later on.

Keep it adjusted! Contrary reasoning makes everything dreary and terrible. Positive thinking envisions anything, whether practical or not, regardless of whether it's identified with the occasion or not. A few people do this by citing superb (irrelevant) Scriptures whenever someone specifies a pessimistic event.

Concentrate on the positive! That is not positive reasoning!

There is a period for misery and understanding the present actualities. It's about how you manage it. Assuming that you don't accomplish something great isn't contrary reasoning. It's assessing life and how to improve it for yourself.

To cite the above book once more: "Positive reasoning just puts a hole between where you are physically and where you figure you "should" be. There are no "should" to a dangerous disease. You'll be more joyful and likely recuperate quicker, if you let go of the same number of should as you can... It took a ton of contrary reasoning - decades now and again - to expedite a sickness. For what reason should up to 14 days of positive thinking dispose of it?"

Compromise with intelligence somewhere close to the sewer and the mists. Concentrate on the positive, however, make it genuine. Your mind and body know the distinction. Health doesn't come without accepting what you think and state. Your account won't trust the amazing.

# Dealing with Negative Thoughts

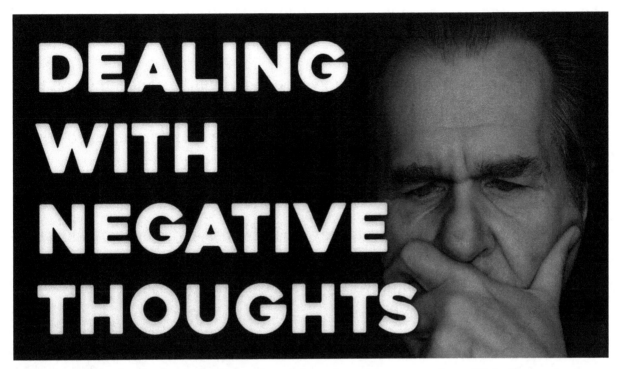

We, as a whole, have negative considerations on occasion. This is typical. For the individuals who experience the ill effects of specific anxiety disorders, contrary reasoning can prompt the beginning of anxiety assaults. When these assaults happen, the individual's satisfaction endures significantly.

The issue with anxiety disorders and contrary reasoning is that one negative idea will regularly form into a progression of all the more dominant negative contemplations. These musings are frequently founded on self-analysis and can lead the individual to trust that the individual in question is by one way or another, not precisely other individuals.

Contrary reasoning, can be controlled once the individual learns a couple of systems. Once leveled out, the individual can start to carry on with an ordinary life once more.

A part of the habits where that you can manage contrary reasoning, which thus can change your conduct, incorporate utilizing strategy known as care.

This is an ancient technique that shows the individual to concentrate on his or her environment and sentiments without being judgmental about either. With this system, there is no set-in stone, fortunate or unfortunate, positive or negative. Things are just what they are, and that's it.

The individual figures out how to stay away from contrary reasoning so that it likewise quiets the nerves and anticipate fits of anxiety. Rather than centering of what is troubling you, you focus on nonpartisan or positive considerations concerning the issue.

The goal behind this strategy isn't to permit the event of negative musings which, as we probably are aware, feed into increasingly negative considerations. By ceasing the cycle from the get-go, you can limit or wipe out anxiety manifestations. It likewise shows you how to abstain from deciding for yourself too cruelly when such judgment isn't justified.

You may likewise profit by utilizing confirmations. These are sure explanations that you rehash to yourself a few times for the day. These positive explanations are particularly valuable when negative idea examples are a danger. Your certifications can be altered to fit any need, whenever.

Both of these strategies enable you to recover control of your manner of thinking. You don't need to endure contrary reasoning if you don't wish it. The key is to supplant negative contemplations with positive considerations.

At whatever point you end up speculation negative contemplations, battle back with positive considerations or attestations. These rehashed positive musings or words will help change your point of view toward the circumstance you are in. You can even keep a diary of your contemplations and scribble down which attestations worked best for a specific issue.

Both of these strategies require practice and will take some an opportunity to ace. In any case, since they are so incredible and compelling, they merit the speculation. They can enable you to carry on with a more joyful life.

You can see an abundance of data on both of these systems either on the web or disconnected. It is your life, take control of it today.

**Step by step instructions to Cope with Anxiety Disorders - Harnessing the Power of the Mind.**

What goes on in your mind impacts how you see and identify with yourself and your general surroundings? Put at the end of the day: What you believe is the thing that you feel and carry on. A lot of research has built up that if you are colonized by contrary reasoning; at that point, this might be reflected in low confidence, anxiety disorders, and wretchedness. The causal impact of contrary thinking is robust to the point that anxiety disorders have been marked by individual scientists as 'mistakes in learning.'

Furthermore, the connection between contrary reasoning and anxiety disorders may take a very long time to advance. For instance, there are numerous individuals out there who experience the ill effects of anxiety disorders because of the maltreatment they encounter as kids. Such abuse undermined their feeling of self-esteem; denied them of their certainty and caused in them the inclination to question everything and everyone.

There is a broad scope of negative or distorted contemplations that anxiety issue sufferers battle with. A first fundamental advance in your endeavor to adapt to anxiety disorders is to investigate your reasoning and attempt and recognize your negative considerations. The following are a couple of kinds of negative contemplations that individuals with anxiety disorders may battle with.

The dread of objection: People with an intemperate terror of being disliked by others become excessively touchy to analysis. Their satisfaction lays on the significant conclusions of others. They firmly want to keep others upbeat. They may think that it is hard to disapprove the requests of others. Their own needs turned out to be optional to the need to win the endorsement.

Mental sifting: This happens when an individual tends to harp and ruminate on small negative parts of even the best circumstance and utilize such pessimism to pass unfriendly judgment on oneself. For instance, after a prospective employee meeting, one may stress that he failed to meet expectations since he didn't address one of the inquiries agreeable to him. This might be regardless of the way that the question was not so significant contrasted with the nine others that he addressed skillfully. The individual may then start to see himself as a washout as a result of that one inquiry.

Mind perusing: This is a case whereby you make decisions about what other individuals are thinking with no proof. For instance, you may infer that someone doesn't care for you or he supposes he is superior to you.

Mind perusers can have relationship issues since they turned out to be excessively suspicious and doubtful of others.

Over-speculation: Here, one mistake is seen as an example of blunders or errors. For instance, after pounding his vehicle in a mishap, the negative individual may reason that he never does anything appropriately and is a terrible driver.

The entire thought of distinguishing negative musings that influence you as anxiety disorders sufferers is with the goal that you can battle and be free of them. Intellectual Behavioral Therapy gives a well-ordered guide on how to fight contrary reasoning and take out anxiety disorders. On my webpage, you will see, on for all intents and purposes each page, connections to online usual treatment suppliers. The vast majority of these treatments depend on humane cognitive treatment. Intellectual conduct treatment treats anxiety disorders more viable than medications.

# How to Discard Negativity

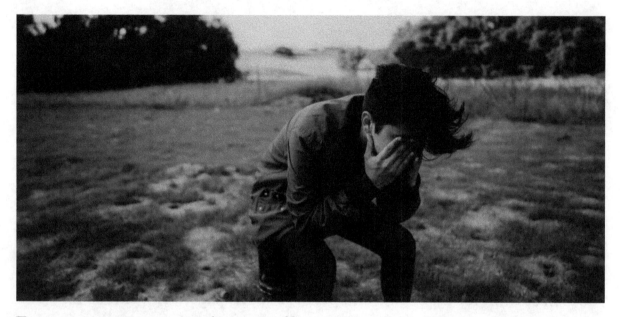

Extreme, contrary reasoning can offer ascent to harmful practices and uninterested attitude when looked with difficulties. As opposed to remaining in favor of the opposite rationale, it is smarter to focus on all the positive things throughout everyday life, be grateful with what you as of now have and monitor your feelings.

We all may have at some time experienced multi-day where nothing appears to go right. This could be very ordinary, yet if you have a feeling that your terrible days are going on more frequently and that the entire world is by all accounts singling out you, the opportunity has already come and gone for you to switch those negative considerations!

**The negative side of contrary reasoning**

Our brain is amazing and can altogether impact our idea of how life ought to be, our practices, and even our odds of making progress. If your psyche is continually harping on the negative part of things, this can have a considerable haul sway on how you see and adapt to difficulties just as how you handle troublesome circumstances. After some time, you may build up a sentiment of weakness, low self-assurance, erratic feelings, and other harmful practices.

Dangerous contrary reasoning can likewise offer ascent to extreme pressure and much different stress-related infirmities, for example, hypertension, burdensome scatters, apprehension, heart issue, weight gain, and a large group of various problems. Concentrate demonstrates that antagonistic individuals have a 20% higher danger of biting the dust and their mind works uniquely in contrast to progressively positive individuals!

## The positive side of positive reasoning

On the other hand, positive reasoning can prompt sentiments of wellbeing, self-strengthening, self-assurance, and a higher likelihood to be effective, remain cheerful, and to be satisfied. Justifiably, it might be hard to change to positive reasoning, particularly when you're confronting emotional difficulties, or you're experiencing weights from all bearings that test you as far as possible. In any case, with practice and persistence, you'll see it isn't too hard to even consider trading your contrary reasoning for positive.

## Here are four different ways to dispose of cynicism:

Be a confident person and spotlight on the constructive. Being a hopeful person isn't tied in with ignoring the contrary things or undesirable minutes throughout everyday life - however remembering them and searching forward for better what might be on the horizon. When was experiencing a predicament, think about all the positive ways you could manage them that will lead you to a satisfactory arrangement.

Practice thankfulness. Be appreciative with what you've just got, and this will lead you to have an uplifting mentality. This will likewise redirect your idea from being negative and instead search out circumstances in the things you as of now have. By rehearsing appreciation, you take conscious of the considerable number of things you're thankful about or even your accomplishments, whether colossal or modest. These can be anything from having a glad family and many dear companions to that business target you've accomplished. It could likewise be your first job advancement, the occasional break you genuinely appreciated or even when you're stranded when an outsider made a special effort to enable you to out.

Be informed about embracing current circumstances. It's anything but difficult to get snared in your daily schedule, and this can weigh vigorously on you, and making you neglect to think on the positive. At the point when gotten up to speed in this circumstance, take a couple of minutes to live in the 'present.' Practice slow and profound breathings and drench yourself in the earth with your faculties. Feel the breeze interacting with your skin, feel the warm contact of your attire on your skin, value the plenitude air encompassing you that offers life to each living thing. This activity is about substantial mindfulness, which can be similarly connected to mental mindfulness. By having spiritual mindfulness, you're better ready to handle any issue continuously.

Cut out the negative winding. Stalling out in rush hour gridlock or in light of the fact that your accomplice has taken your vehicle without letting you know, is by all accounts a typical response, however it's hugely a misuse of your vitality (other than ruining your positive state of mind) to get warmed up over something you can't control. It's okay to be irate. However, it isn't, if you allow your terrible inclination to remain for the remainder of your day. Disclose to yourself that however, you're troubled about it, yet you'll figure out how to get over this. For example, move in tuning in to the music or tunes while you're stuck in rush hour gridlock. In like manner, advise yourself that your accomplice could be in some crisis to have taken your vehicle in such a surge. All the more significantly, ask yourself this: Is the circumstance worth getting me worried up and makes me age quicker? When it isn't, at that point, leave the issue for what it's worth or forget about it.

# 6 Benefits to Natural Treatments for Panic Disorder

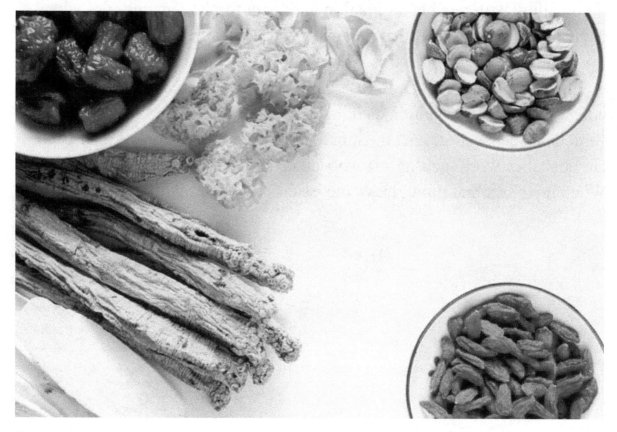

Psychological, social treatment is generally acknowledged and has turned into the treatment of decision for uneasiness and frenzy issue. It is evaluated that around 80-85% of individuals lead an assault-free life after finishing their humane treatment sessions.

CBT centers around two fundamental viewpoints with the first being recognizing and subsequently changing the negative reasoning examples that lead to the uneasiness and frenzy. The second part of CBT for frenzy issue is to desensitize the experience through the compelling introduction of what is dreaded. Intellectual conduct treatment fundamentally changes how you think, and in this way, how you respond to whatever the upgrades are that instigates your tension.

The most critical advantage to CBT as an appropriate treatment to frenzy issue is the way that you will probably carry on with your life assault free. Anyway, other similarly incredible advantages will enable you to lead all the more satisfying life!

**1. Figuring out how to smoothly address fears:** Panic assaults can be depicted as a nonsensical response to a dread, memory, occasion, place, and so forth. It is a strong response to the psyches error of said occasions. While the feeling itself might be legitimate, the disastrous response to it regularly isn't. For instance, numerous individuals have a dread of suffocating, yet an individual who experiences a frenzy issue may encounter a severe response to this dread while remaining in a puddle of water. CBT will show you how to smoothly and securely address these apprehensions.

**2. Compelling Stress Management:** let's be straightforward - most grown-ups could gain proficiency with some things about successfully dealing with their feelings of anxiety, so you aren't allowed here! In any case, it tends to be said that an individual who experiences nervousness issue has an even lower pressure limit. Where the average individual thinks about a disappointing occasion while considering other factors, you may go into full worry mode. The impacts of weight on the body is so harming, rationally - as well as physically too. So, carrying on with a real existence where you are always pushed, or very nearly stress is counterproductive to your wellbeing.

**3. Expanded Self-Esteem:** Panic assaults can be humiliating for the sufferer. Because of the absence of extensive information about the confusion, many experiences this issue alone. They trust that something isn't right with them or that individuals will chuckle at them once they know the reality. As a result, they may maintain a strategic distance from open communication and socialization. By figuring out how to smoothly address your feelings of dread, and deal with your feelings of anxiety - you will recover the certainty you should be that cherishing and the intuitive individual you want!

**4. Lower Depression:** Panic issue can be a disengaging condition for somebody who feels misjudged, disliked, and not quite the same as the rest. These emotions can cause profound episodes of wretchedness. So, diminishing that wretchedness is a natural reaction when you conquer your feelings of dread, increment confidence, and learn compelling pressure the executives.

**5. Turn around contrary reasoning and propensities:** It is regularly said that we are the cause all our problems. Our contrary thinking and unfortunate propensities cause pointless torment and anguish in our lives. This is even doubly so for an individual experiencing nervousness issue. Indeed, this is generally the underlying driver of the clutters. Freeing yourself of the contrary reasoning is principal to your accomplishment in defeating your assaults!

**6. Full investment in YOUR life!** Imagine what it will feel like once you start to carry on with your life free of dread and fits of anxiety! You will pick up significant serenity, the capacity to go where you need - when you need, you'll discharge that people person somewhere within you that is merely asking to get out! You will at long last have the option to carry on with your life, not only exist in it!

Intellectual conduct treatment is viewed as the best fix to uneasiness and frenzy issue - and there's a valid justification for this which is basically: It works!

# Why Negative Thoughts Can Be So Destructive

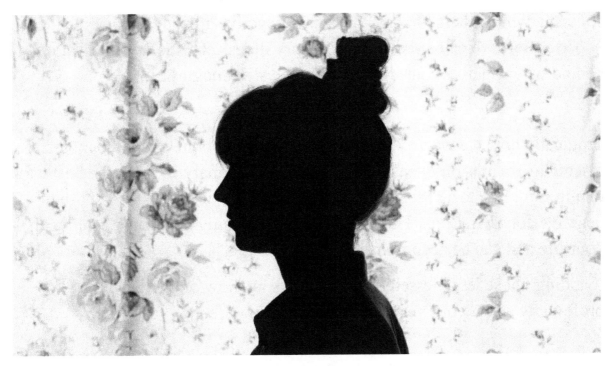

Everybody has a decision on concerning how they think yet, as a rule, we are managed by pessimism, and numerous individuals still don't understand why negative contemplations can be so damaging.

It is antagonism that achieves tension and misery and if not controlled, can abbreviate your future. Discouragement can assimilate you and even though your specialist could endorse medicine for it, would you genuinely like to carry on with an incredible remainder on antidepressants? Depending taking drugs can influence you rationally separated from the symptoms that frequently goes with any medicine.

No one but you can control your contemplations and when you proceed with the way of pessimism your satisfaction will radically fall apart.

Negative considerations start with the stress of what may transpire to seeing others improvement and achieve their objectives. This like this will instigate covetousness and envy because your life has stayed static, simply enduring while others prosper. It is these negative attributes that expedite hypertension, which can result in coronary illness. This is one motivation behind why negative considerations can be so damaging.

Tragically how the world is today with everything done dangerously fast, discouragement is on the expansion, as is the coronary illness. The best way to quit turning into a casualty of this cutting-edge disease is to dispose of negative considerations. This is finished by focusing on such is positive in your life and can be accomplished.

In aiding, those less blessed than yourself somehow or another can profoundly affect your very own reasoning and life.

You need to take a gander at the rundown of philanthropies that well-known individuals buy into which encourages you to understand that stress and anguish are wholly lost. When you witness, individuals biting the dust of ailment and starvation in numerous pieces of the world, the lowering impact this without a doubt has, ought to motivate anybody to escape their negative attitude.

Kathrynn's goal is to share her insight and encounters experienced during a troublesome life in which she stood up to mental pitilessness, bringing about an absence of confidence and worth.

Even though it has required investment to survive, she has had the option to proceed onward to an actual existence of euphoria and motivation and together with her significant other, Mark, they have joined their background bringing about helping other people in similar conditions.

**Step by step instructions to Overcome Negative Thoughts - Reformatting Your Unconscious Mind.**

Negative musings carry bothersome outcomes to our lives. It is one of the most significant obstructions that we have that made us quit seeking after our fantasies. It can likewise be merely the motivation behind why we need certainty and we some of the time don't have confidence in ourselves. If you need to transform yourself into the better, read on for specific tips on the most proficient method to conquer negative considerations and begin to carry on with a superior and more joyful life.

Negative considerations, particularly those that have been modified profoundly into our intuitive can gigantically influence our frames of mind towards things and our convictions too. We are frequently reluctant to catch a few open doors towards progress since we regularly figure we don't have a clue how to do it, or we adversely think we are not very keen to do it. We dread remaining before the open since we figure we may commit an error and we dread that individuals may giggle at us.

These negative examples of musings are among those that ruin us to be cheerful and, yet it isn't up to where it is possible to change that. You can figure out how to defeat negative contemplations and change your reasoning to something that can do you all the more magnificent. Here are a couple of systems.

## Positive confirmations

Positive confirmations are short positive explanations that you let yourself know over and again. By rehashing it frequently, it will help drive these positive contemplations where it counts into your intuitive and dispense with those negative ones. You can do this by playing a video or sound of positive proclamations that you tune in to every day or each morning. Tuning in to positive musings every day will steadily enable you to dispose of negative ones and follow up on the positive explanations that you have for yourself.

## Contemplation and perception

Contemplation is an old practice. However, it has additionally helped such vast numbers of individuals in the advanced occasions to manage pressure, improve fixation and center, and restore their bodies from physical and mental strength. Contemplation utilizes positive musings too, and that helps a great deal in calming your psyche and in putting positive considerations into your intuitive. Perception causes you to reconstruct your brain also to consider positive things and imagine yourself in favorable circumstances to dispose of negative ones.

It is significant excessively that if you need to figure out how to conquer negative musings with reflection or perception, you need to rehearse them routinely, and you need to figure out how to do it accurately so you will likewise receive great rewards from this old practice.

## Mesmerizing

Self-mesmerizing is likewise a mainstream approach to separate those negative considerations that have been developed in your subliminal for a long time since you were a youngster. Negative contemplations are once in a while challenging to dispose of, and it might require you to connect with your subliminal to have the option to reconstruct your psyche and your reasoning.

By spellbinding, or self-trance, you can give your mind some sleep-inducing recommendations that will help a great deal in supplanting negative musings with positive ones. Hypnotherapy has been utilized in therapeutic science to enable people to diminish the torment and furthermore used in numerous applications particularly in conquering trepidation and injury, which are pessimistic contemplations that have been in our intuitive personality for a long time.

Become familiar with these couple of systems on the most proficient method to beat contrary contemplations, what's more, you will, over the long haul, watch a more straightforward way to be a positive, increasingly fruitful and a lot more joyful individual.

# CHAPTER FOUR
## Healing Negative Thoughts and Feelings with Gemstone Medicine

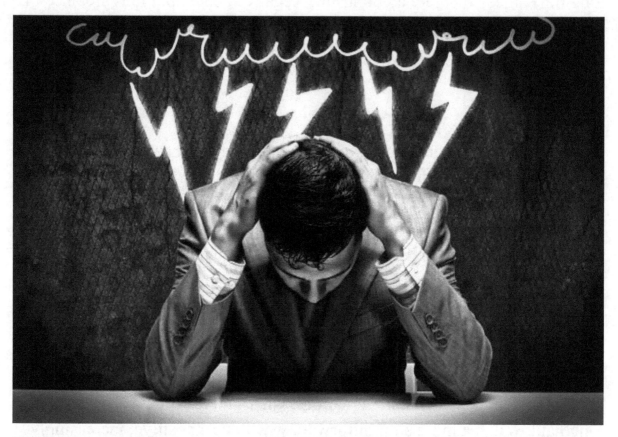

When you have a sickness, regardless of whether it's a common cold or a hazardous ailment, it isn't extraordinary to feel uneasiness, bitterness, sadness, and even anger about your condition. You may stress over the work you can't do, be frightful of up and coming therapeutic strategies or guesses or feel baffled when you miss exercises with family and companions. These negative considerations and emotions add to the seriousness of the physical issue and draw out recuperation. The more you stress, worry, and envision the most exceedingly terrible, the harder it will be to recuperate.

Drawn out negative contemplations and emotions you may have about sickness or damage will gather in your emanation. They resemble barriers and hinder typical inflows of the mending life power from achieving your body. They can likewise keep your body from giving up the unwanted energies related to sickness and damage. This can propagate a condition or exacerbate it. Moreover, negative contemplations and sentiments initially brought forth from a disease cured sometime in the past, can wait for an incredible duration. Their quality in your emanation can make you powerless to different sorts of ailment or damage.

If you build up a propensity for communicating particular negative contemplations and sentiments, they can begin to influence physical tissue. Once tied down in your body, they will in general solidify and fix tissue. They have contracted tissue limits bloodstream to the region, thus denying it organic supplements and the robust framework's white blood cells. Such tissue winds up got dried out and confine the capacity of lymph vessels from taking up and expelling poisons and cell squanders.

The physical impacts of negative musings and feelings are predominant in our general public. For instance, when the negative articulations related to pressure become tied down in the body, they can bunch muscles in the shoulders and back, prompting neck and back torment. They can show as aggregations of plaque inside the supply routes, causing arteriosclerosis. They can likewise fix the stomach, upsetting processing and causing indigestion malady.

Much of the time, the physical body can conquer the disease. The negative considerations and feelings wait to compound future conditions-except if they are dealt with legitimately.

For the most part, we consider recuperating as far as physical tissue. Our outlooks, frames of mind, and feelings should likewise be amended to stop their negative surge.

Present day drug does not address the psychological and enthusiastic donors of sick wellbeing, other than to recognize worry as a dominant causative factor or send you to a therapist. Conversely, gemstone vitality prescription not just perceives the destructive impact of negative considerations and sentiments, however, causes you to kill them, let go of them, and evacuate them, so they never again contaminate your emanation.

Gemstone vitality prescription comprises of gemstone apparatuses, in particular, therapeutic gemstone pieces of jewelry, gemstone medication cures that are taken orally, and gemstone treatment, which is connected in the air by a gemstone treatment expert.

When you wear restorative gemstone accessories, their energies transmit into your quality to frequently adjust, explain, and inspire enthusiastic and mental powers. It ends up simpler to perceive negative contemplations and emotions. Your psyche and feelings will likewise draw upon the gemstones' strengths for solidarity to give up the constant examples associated with negative articulations. It will be simpler to supplant negative considerations and feelings with positive ones.

Gemstone pieces of jewelry that can enable you to mend your psyche and feelings incorporate rhodonite, which balances out dispersed and imbalanced emotions, and rose quartz, whose vitality ousts and discharge passionate energies that have penetrated your body, and energizes a more beneficial progression of sanitized feelings. What's more, sodalite absorbs and kills the billows of negative considerations that dirty your atmosphere, hinder your brain, and make you feel troubled. It can likewise discharge negative idea shapes that have held up in your body and that disturb work and propagate illness. Pieces of jewelry that contain purple rainbow fluorite are useful in separating the constraining propensities and examples that sustain negative outpourings, also, this gemstone encourages open your attention to these examples with the goal that you can assume better responsibility for yourself.

Helpful gemstone neckbands are perfect for working legitimately with your brain and feelings, and for killing and clearing the buildup of negative contemplations and emotions from your air. When they influence physical tissue in any capacity, causing any side effects, it's an ideal opportunity to take an oral gemstone prescription cure, which discharges recuperating gemstone vitality legitimately to your cells.

A gemstone drug cure called Energy Clearing expels and scatters the contamination deserted by negative contemplations and feelings. When you take this gemstone medication, it begins working inside your body at the cell level. This cure raises the vibrations of your cells, which expands their bioelectric turn, so they usually pushed off undesirable mental and enthusiastic energies. The Energy Clearing cure likewise causes your body to discharge and scatter unwanted energies related to contamination and sickness, in this manner helping you mend physically, as well.

Gemstone advisors pursue different conventions and utilize various methods to apply gemstones in your emanation to treat the psychological and passionate contamination that might gather there. Gemstone treatment gives all of you the advantages of wearing gemstone pieces of jewelry, but since the gemstones are connected powerfully, and with center and aim, results are accomplished much sooner.

Restorative gemstone pieces of jewelry and gemstone drug cures are perfect. You can wear gemstone pieces of jewelry while taking gemstone drug. Moreover, both can be utilized alongside homegrown or pharmaceutical prescriptions to adjust and finish your mending routine. Gemstone treatment uses the two pieces of jewelry and cures and offers the best help for mending your contemplations and feelings, so they have less of an effect on your physical wellbeing. Gemstones won't do practically everything for you. It additionally takes a craving to improve yourself, self-restraint to pick positive contemplations and emotions, and self-esteem to excuse your old ways and acknowledge more current, more advantageous articulations.

**Controlling Your Negative Thoughts**

Vast numbers of us are blameworthy of reasoning contrarily; however, we are not entirely mindful of the harm contrary thinking can have on our wellbeing. Controlling your negative contemplations ought to be defeated before it spirals and takes you to the profundities of despondency.

It is one of the first drivers of discouragement and some psychological instabilities. If not controlled, sadness has been known to lead a few people to end it all. Since gloom is so necessary, today specialists are endorsing medications to battle the ailment, and now and again, patients are ignorant of the unwanted reactions and the harm that can be caused. As a rule, the appropriate response lies with you, not through medicine. It is a lot simpler to control your negative contemplations than set out upon a protracted course of medications, joined by upsetting symptoms.

We as a whole face affliction in our lives; however, the mystery is to gain from it and not sink into a condition of despair because of it. Cynicism is irresistible, and if you encircle yourself with similarly invested individuals, it will have a significant adverse effect without anyone else thinks. Moreover, the more constructive individuals that you partner with, the more positive you can turn into. Consequently, it is to your most significant advantage to mingle more with this kind of individual.

By concentrating on all the beneficial things throughout your life and being appreciative for all that nature accommodates you, it can assist you with beginning controlling your negative considerations. In aiding those less lucky than yourself, everything can be put into viewpoint as far as you could tell. We underestimate such a significant amount in our lives yet saving an idea for debilitated youngsters, and those individuals kept to a wheel seat or malignancy sufferers then you clearly should remember you're good fortune and acknowledge that your life isn't so awful all things considered.

Numerous well-known individuals dedicate a great deal of their time visiting and aiding those less blessed than themselves. On the odd event when a superstar is talked with, for the most part, say that they have a lot to be grateful for in their life and this is their method for returning something. So why not expect to take a comparable activity?

# How to Remove a Negative Thought from Your Mind

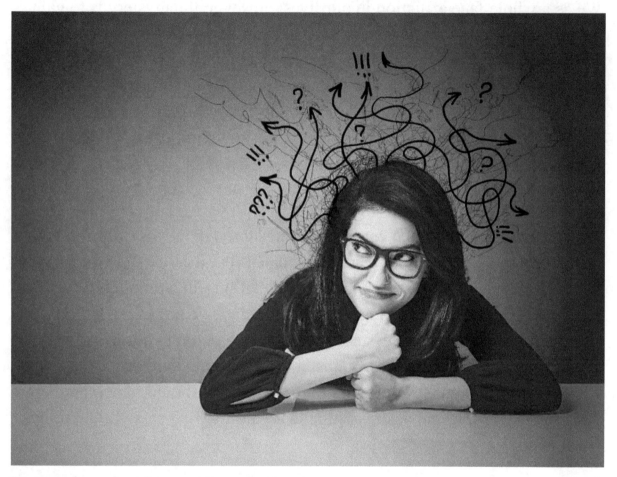

**Recognize what is most imperative to you**

Before you can begin to effectively take a shot at your considerations and expelling the negative musings from your mind, you should first be sure about what is most essential to you in your life. By recognizing what is most significant, you will at that point have the option to comprehend and realize what you have to do to guarantee that the changing of your musings will profit you over the long haul. Without understanding what is most imperative to you your capacity to know whether thinking is harmful or not is altogether influenced.

## Comprehend your objectives

You likewise need an unmistakable comprehension of your objectives in life altogether for the reworking of negative musings to profit you however much as could reasonably be expected. When you have a clear and all-around characterized objective you are moving towards you can alter your contemplations to guarantee they are in the best arrangement with your intentions as could be allowed. You can't adequately change a negative idea to a real impression except if you know where the plan needs to lead you.

## Investigate your present contemplations

Before you can start to expel your negative contemplations and supplant them with elegantly composed new positive considerations, you should first realize what your musings are and choose if the present reflections you have are either negative or positive. This is exceptionally easy to do. Every 20 or 30 minutes, have an essential alert go off on your telephone or PC that you will use as a trigger to record your considerations. When you are recording these considerations, don't pass judgment on the off chance that they are fortunate or unfortunate positive or negative. When causing the rundown to do only that, make a rundown.

It is merely after you have dealt with structure this rundown for a couple for a considerable length of time that you return to the full review and begin to pass judgment on each idea as being absolute or negative. The key here isn't to pass an examination on it dependent on the wording, judge it dependent on what is most essential to you and your objectives. On the off chance that the thinking is an arrangement with what is most imperative to you AND additionally causes you to progress towards your goals, at that point, this is a definite idea and one you need to keep. Put these positive contemplations in a rundown and read those favorable and advantageous musings day by day. If an idea in your unique outline either does not coordinate what is most essential to you or potentially positively move you towards your objectives, then these are negative musings. These negative contemplations go into an alternate rundown, which we will work with straightaway.

**Change the negative into positive to coordinate your objectives.**

Preceding working with the negative musings makes sure to peruse and concentrating on the positive contemplations your record. This will fortify these positive musings and begin to fill space in your psyche with these positive contemplations significantly progressively then they were at that point there. Presently the time has come to take a gander at your rundown of negative considerations. You have two options you can make about each idea.

When the idea has positively no reference what so ever to either what is most imperative to you or move you towards your objectives, at that point, dispose of them. Compose these unbeneficial considerations onto little bits of paper, begin a low flame in a flame pit or a BBQ barbecue, and to discharge these musings perpetually, toss them into the fire and ensure they copy totally.

The remainder of your negative contemplations rundown may have something that is an arrangement with what is most imperative to you or associated with your objectives. This is the place you get the chance to take this negative idea and change it, so it is currently both positive and in arrangement with both what is most imperative to you and your objectives.

Take as much time as fundamental while doing this since you need to guarantee the new musings you are putting into your mind are sure and an arrangement with both of the two classifications f what is most significant and your objectives.

**Six Tips for Turning Negative Thoughts into Positive Ones**

Regardless of how positive you are, there is likely in any event one negative inclination or believed that wet blankets into your psyche once a day. Negative contemplations have numerous birthplaces. They can create from not feeling admirable, encountering low confidence, or questioning one's self. Considering the way this happens to everybody, how do a few people seem, by all accounts, to be progressively fruitful at transforming pessimistic contemplations into constructive ones preceding the antagonism becomes and winds up counterproductive? This section gives a few hints on squelching negative musings before they get an opportunity to decompose and eject.

1. At the point when a negative idea comes into your head, pause for a moment to comprehend and evaluate where it is coming from. On the off chance that it is an issue or issue that you have power over, take a couple of minutes, and build up a system to determine it. On the off chance that you can't control the issue or issue, acknowledge it to the best degree conceivable and proceed onward. You would prefer not to invest energy being negative over things in which you have no control.

2. At the point when negative considerations creep into your head, recognize them for what they are. Investigate all aspects of the negative contemplations, as you might most likely gain from them. Maybe the negative musings are giving a chance to distinguish and investigate

potential answers for an issue or issue. We regularly gain most from encountering and working through adverse circumstances or saw disappointments.

3. Build up a rundown of positive insistences and post them in an area where you see them every day, for example, your washroom or kitchen. Audit these insistences first thing toward the beginning of the day and just before you hit the hay. This should assist you with positively starting your day and help you to unwind at night. Build up a rundown of certifications that is one of a kind to you; one that mirrors your qualities, gifts, abilities, qualities, properties, and those things for which you are generally appreciative. When you center around positive thoughts, the negative ones will have less of a chance to attack your musings.

4. Disapprove of negative emotions and musings. You have to understand that you do have authority over how you feel about individuals, circumstances, and occasions. In this way, regardless of the amount, someone insults you or how terrible the thing was, attempt to abstain from giving it a chance to affect you negatively. Vent, take a full breath and turn your considerations to positive ones. Your day will be significantly improved if you do.

So, whenever a negative idea creeps into your brain, consider where it may originate from an attempt to gain from it. Give it the time it needs yet abstain from dwelling on it. Endeavor to change over negative musings into positive ones as fast as could be expected under the circumstances, build up a rundown of confirmations and survey them day by day, help yourself to remember those things for which you are thankful every day, and discover that you can transform negative contemplations into positive ones, as you are the person who has extreme command over your considerations and sentiments.

# Tips for How to Stop Worrying

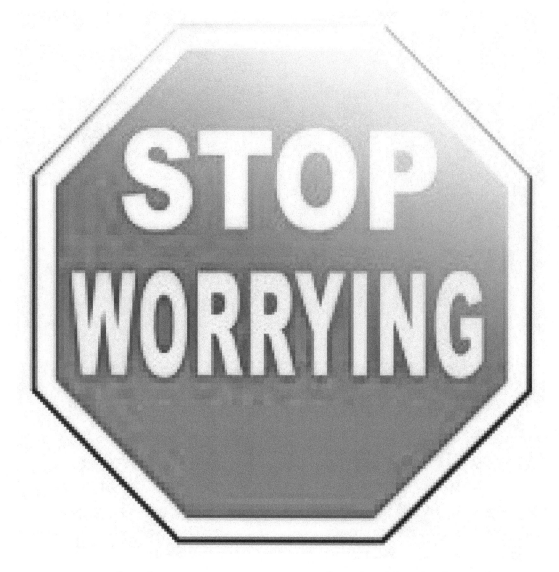

Stress can control as long as you can remember, and it can harm how you see the contrasts between dream and reality. Everyone, to some degree, may be apprehensive about supporting their activity in this economy or attempting to prop a relationship up, however, you can likewise demolish yourself by sending an excess of consideration concentrated on these things.

People may fall back on stressing over their professional stability, because of an inclination that they have no power over the issue. However, in all actuality, you can assume responsibility for this circumstance by evaluating your present arrangement of abilities and achievements, and you may choose to gain ground in your training with the target of an increasingly secure business circumstance.

These sorts of things will help you by improving your confidence in yourself, and enable you to collaborate with individuals you didn't at first know. Supplanting your relationship stresses with more excellent quality time and creating more grounded bonds with your cherished one can lighten those anxieties.

Another progression making progress toward ceasing stress is to share the issue, and although this may not be a speedy arrangement, it'll help to calm the anxiety. Is your worry because of a dread of some mysterious circumstance? If so, handling this situation legitimately is the thing that I propose to figure out How to Stop Worrying about it.

For example, you may have dread about skydiving, which would be fine when you were going to skydive, yet if not, at that point you can delete this stress by reminding your mind that you'll not ever bounce from a plane, this way, this is an additional concern.

Figuring out How to Stop Worrying enables you to figure out how to manage the things that you can modify, because there are a lot of certifiable worries for us every day. If you have had negative encounters previously, and this can change how you manage circumstances, you may need to look later on.

Getting all worked up over something isn't sound, and when the occasion happens you, for the most part, find that there was nothing genuine to stress over in any case. This is valid, perceiving how to quit stressing involves how you set yourself up for specific occasions. When you dispose of conceivably adverse outcomes from your activities, you can anticipate positive results.

You can rehearse this with your companions as you're figuring out how to quit stressing. Concentrate on excellent outcomes, and you'll start to comprehend the least challenging course through these sorts of circumstances. A mentor that can assist you with fundamental abilities, or chatting with individuals who have encountered the situations you stress over, can likewise be useful.

You ought to likewise abstain from utilizing medications or liquor to enable you to manage dread and stress. These things can improve your feelings and give you a sentiment of powerlessness. When you center around positive creatures that are controllable, such as remaining fit and reliable, your stresses will appear to be little and inconsequential, and may even vanish in the plan of things.

**Ways on How to Stop Worrying**

While it is legitimate to see stress as a useful human response to danger, an excess of stressing can clear route for some destructive impacts. The weakening impacts of highlighting rise when it as of now leaves hand. It can cause an assortment of effects on your physical and mental prosperity in straightforward ways.

Subsequently, such essential impacts can cause out and out uneasiness issue; these will likewise decline the specific tension issue that you may as of now have. You ought to dependably screen yourself; particularly when you as of now stress excessively, pointlessly.

If you end up in a consistent condition of stress, don't postpone on utilizing measures that will address the issue. Try not to give the unnecessary stressing lead to a nervousness a chance to clutter; or if you as of now experience the ill effects of one, abstain from fueling and fortifying the turmoil. It is never too early to be free from tension. The more you develop it, the steadier it moves toward becoming, and the more profound you fall into an endless loop of uneasiness and dread.

To keep the most noticeably awful situation from occurring, one path is to figure out how to quit stressing excessively.

A portion of the viable suggestions on the best way to quit stressing include:

**1. Challenge and control your considerations**

In the wake of recognizing and concentrating on your stresses, begin to break down them coherently. It is safe to say that they are as awful as they appear? What is the most noticeably terrible thing that can leave them? Is it true that they are incredibly worth stressing over? Your justification enables you to check the gravity, or detail, of the circumstance. In case you're in a consistent condition of stress, this usually infers you stress even over the most trivial things, or even non-undermining examples. Testing your considerations and convictions can cause you to understand that a few things are not worth stressing over - that at last, you can deal with the dreaded circumstance, and you will finish up being alright.

## 2. Look for help

Since stressing an excessive amount of has turned into a propensity, you may discover trouble in being sensible towards your stresses. Ask your family and companions to enable you to justify and challenge your contemplations. Tuning in to what others state can support your assurance into being coherent, and into speculation decidedly.

## 3. Exercise, play sports, relax

Stress assumes an exceptional job in stressing excessively. Discover approaches to lessen the pressure. Physical movement can help reduce pressure; it additionally empowers you to redirect your negative contemplations. Thus, relaxation and having a decent rest allows your body to capacity well so as not to wind up inclined to a lot of pressure and nervousness.

In any case, don't stop with merely realizing how to quit stressing. As expressed before, being in a consistent condition of stress is profoundly symptomatic of uneasiness issue, particularly of summed up tension issue. Stressing excessively and tension have circumstances and relevant results interaction with one another; along these lines, you should see whether you as of now experience the ill effects of acute nervousness. If you do, at that point, you should profit yourself of treatment techniques that dispense with it.

Taking out nervousness can be a severe undertaking, yet a remunerating one. Different common treatment strategies are inside your range. Such incredible methods don't occasion warrant the utilization of drugs; subsequently, you won't need to stress of adverse reactions. This is because, without anyone else's input, such common strategies can rapidly and forever wipe out your nervousness. When your uneasiness is gone, you won't need to stress how to quit stressing excessively, once more.

# Step by step instructions to Stop Worrying About Everything: 4 Awesome Tips

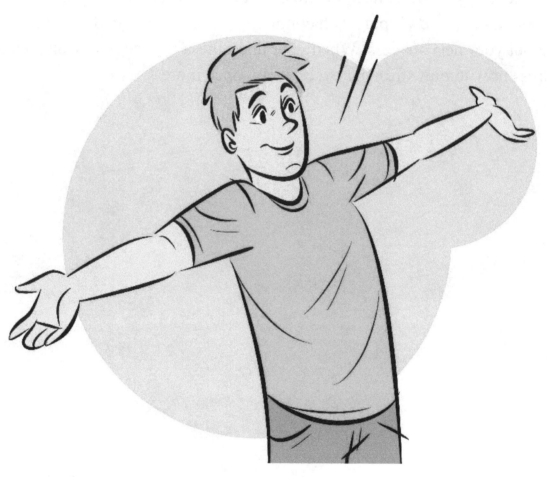

Here and there, we don't have the foggiest idea of how to quit stressing over everything. We can't stop pondering the most pessimistic scenario situations, the what-uncertainties, the negative contemplations, the ceaseless obligations at home and work.

All these keep us up during the evening and take steps to push us over the edge during the day. For what reason do we permit this? In case we're not cautious, stress and stressing can assume control over our lives, making us ineffective, unmotivated and immobilized by dread.

Recapture control of your anxious personality by figuring out how to quit agonizing over everything. Here's the ticket:

## Tip # 1: Accept Uncertainty.

You can't control everything. There will dependably be things or circumstances that won't go your direction. Pondering things that could turn out badly can harm your wellbeing and make you hopeless. Not just that, they can even draw in negative vitality and become inevitable outcomes.

So, don't consider them any longer. Everything will deal with itself at the correct time. Try not to pass up all the beneficial things you have at the present minute.

If you need to figure out how to quit agonizing over everything, you should grapple with the way that you can't generally have assurance in your life; yet understand that you include the power inside you to determine any difficulties you may experience.

## Tip # 2: Delay Your Worries.

Banishing stresses isn't a simple thing, particularly for endless worriers. Instead of smothering your fears (which will, in the long run, reemerge at any rate), figure out how to delay them.

This aide since it shields you from dwelling on them in right now. Ending up better at deferring your stresses likewise encourages you to experience a more prominent feeling of command over yourself and the circumstance.

## Tip # 3: Challenge Your Negative Thoughts.

As a worrier, you regularly make a hasty judgment - you expect that the circumstance will finish up gravely. Try not to describe the world as riskier than it truly is.

When you need to figure out how to quit stressing over everything, you need to begin distinguishing what it is that makes you suspicious. Rather than review them as deterrents that you're confident you can't in any way, shape or form rout, consider them to be difficulties you can survive.

The thing with worriers is that they are disposed of continuously to see the world as half-vacant. Figuring out how to distinguish, inspect, and challenge your negative contemplations will enable you to pick up an increasingly adjusted point of view about your circumstance and why you ought not to stress over it.

## Tip # 4: Relax.

This is most likely the best tip on the best way to quit agonizing over everything. Relax. Taking full breaths and reflecting will support your body and your brain to quiet down.

Keep in mind that you can keep all these pessimism under control as long as you deal with yourself and keep your considerations and feelings in charge.

# How to Stop Worrying About Growing Old

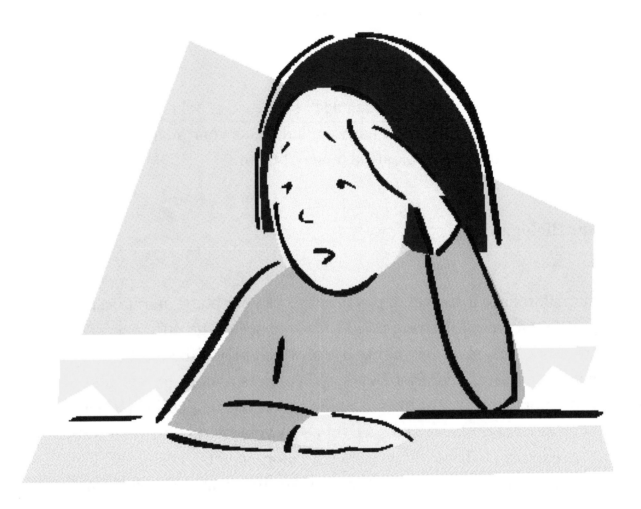

Individuals stress over a wide range of things, and as they get more seasoned many starts to stress over how rapidly their childhood is disappearing. They think that it is hard to acknowledge the way that they are never again youthful, and don't feel as fiery and loaded with life as they once did. In reality, they look in the mirror and see silver hair, wrinkles and hanging cheeks and miracle where all the time went.

In any case, for many, things are not as awful as they may appear. A few people are, actually, much more youthful than their ordered age (the number of years they have lived). What's more, I'm sure you have seen this. They look and act years more youthful than they are. What this lets us know is that individuals have two ages: their ordered age and the actual age. Also, you might be one of the lucky ones with a certain age, much not exactly your ordered age.

How would you decide your exact age? For reasons unknown, it's influenced by two numbers: what we allude to as your nuclear age and your mental age. We should look at each one of them.

**Your Biological Age**

Your natural age is the valid, physical age of your body, and it isn't equivalent to your following period. It is the age of the different frameworks that make up your body, of which two of the most significant are your cardiovascular framework and your respiratory framework. Furthermore, however, it likewise relies upon your endocrine (structures that produce hormones), and such things as your blood glucose level, pulse, and even your cholesterol levels. What's more, maybe most significant, it relies upon your general quality, which thus relies upon the shape and size of your muscles.

It's notable that for the average individual, the real frameworks of their body decline in effectiveness by about 1% every year after age 40. So, by the age of 60, they are 20% less productive. Once more, this doesn't occur to everybody. Exercise has a significant effect; it has been demonstrated that it can lessen the rate by half. What's more, obviously, appropriate eating routine, control of pressure, and getting adequate rest likewise help.

## Mental Age

Your mental age is related to your psyche and is the piece of maturing individuals usually partner with dementia. For it we need to think about three things:

- Distraction
- Capacity to learn and hold new material
- Enthusiastic working
- Distraction

Everybody overlooks things now and again, and there's no uncertainty that it turns out to be increasingly pervasive as we age. A standout amongst the most widely recognized things we overlook is the names of individuals. Somebody discloses to us their name, and after 30 minutes we've forgotten it. What's more, when acne that we go into another space for something, we here and there forget what we went for when we arrive. It's humiliating, and we once in a while shake our head and state to ourselves, "Ugh... another senior minute."

Everybody has these issues are they become more established, and much of the time they are not genuine. An ongoing report has demonstrated that the "dread of memory misfortune" is, in reality, more regrettable than the misfortune itself. It can, truth be told, make you considerably increasingly absent-minded. So, it's best not to get steamed when you overlook sporadically. There are a few purposes behind neglect (other than breaking down mind); among them are stress, diversion, uneasiness, and stress.

## Capacity to Learn Rapidly

Likewise, significant in connection to mental maturing is your capacity to learn, grasp, and hold. Is it in the same class as it used to be? Presumably not. In any case, that isn't an issue, and it's anything but difficult to defeat somewhat. To work getting it done, your cerebrum needs a decent supply of oxygen, and this might be your concern. As I referenced before, the proficiency of your respiratory framework (and your high-impact limit) diminishes as you age, and thus less oxygen gets to your mind. There is a solution to this. Studies have demonstrated that activity can build it all together.

What's more, you should keep your mind dynamic. A portion of the things that help are:

- Perusing
- Working riddles and crosswords
- Diversions that animate the psyche
- Generally, the TV isn't great, yet some programs are useful.
- Passionate Age
- Your passionate age is likewise part of your mental age. It's identified with things, for example,
- Controlling negative considerations
- Remaining calm
- Controlling pressure
- Coexisting with individuals

Unusually, this is one spot where more established individuals every now and again show improvement over their more youthful partners. A dash survey of 340,000 individuals taken a couple of years back demonstrates the accompanying fascinating outcomes:

- Age of most elevated pressure: 25 - 35
- Feelings of anxiety by any significant drop after 50
- Joy is commonly most astounding in the late '60s and mid-'70s (likewise moderately high in youngsters)
- Age most drastically averse to have negative contemplations: 70's and 80's

**What do Older People Worry About?**

**How about we take a gander at a portion of the things:**

- Losing appeal (male pattern baldness, wrinkles, weight gain)
- The dread of the sickness (coronary illness, disease, etc.)
- Dejection
- Misfortune for opportunity
- Passing

Do they look recognizable? Indeed, any of these things are conceivable as you become more established, yet they are not unavoidable, and they don't occur just to more established individuals; they can transpire. There's no uncertainty that illnesses, for example, a cancerous growth, coronary disease, diabetes, and Alzheimer's are progressively underlying in more seasoned individuals. There are many ways you can take to reduce the risks of getting them. You ought to do what you can to lower your opportunity of getting any of the abovementioned and leave it at that. Try not to stress over them... yet, how would you quit stressing?

**Step by step instructions to Stop Worrying**

So, what do we do? Start by recollecting the well-known adage, "age is only a number." Take it to heart. The main thing that truly matters is how old you feel. Undoubtedly, a 23 - years learn at Miami, and Yale Universities demonstrated that individuals who had a favorable view of maturing (and acknowledged their identity) lived on the average, 7.5 years longer than the individuals who did not.

How you feel about your age has a significant effect on your wellbeing, joy, and even your life span. Getting old is a piece of life, and all things considered, it's something you need to figure out how to acknowledge. Stress will exacerbate it. Concentrate instead on stuff you appreciate. Look for new experiences; keep occupied with things you want to do. Focus on them - not your absence of youth. Make an effort not to try and consider it. An inspirational frame of mind is, and this implies at whatever point negative musings enter your account you ought to dispose of them right away. Substitute a definite idea for them.

Acting youthful likewise helps (yet don't go over the edge). Without a doubt, acting and feeling youthful makes you look younger. What's more, recollect that you will feel younger if you practice the four unique things that will expand your life:

- Exercise (30 to 40 minutes every day)
- Decrease pressure
- Appropriate sustenance and diet (eat less and better)
- Adequate rest.
- Different things that likewise help are:
- Get out and mingle
- Music (sing, play a melodic instrument, or tune in)

# How to Stop Worrying - The Hardest Habit to Break

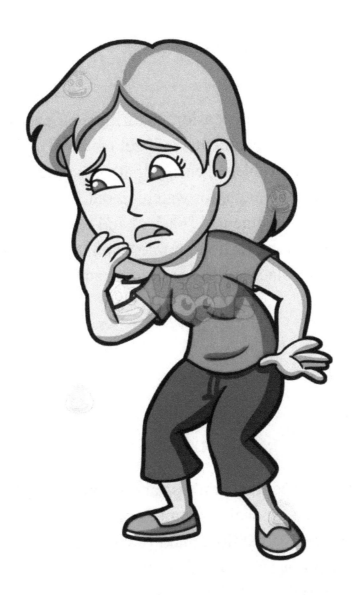

The appropriate response is - you can't. There, what number of individuals will say that? The fact of the matter is that everyone worries - that's right; nobody is safe. Do you know, I've heard that even somebody as renowned as Woody Allen is inclined to a wrinkled temple every so often. Kidding separated, a touch of stress from time to time is certifiably not an awful thing - it demonstrates you're alive and working. When you stress unnecessarily, it can turn into a hard propensity to break, and the issue ought to be tended to before it winds up unmanageable. So here goes with a couple of thoughts on the most proficient method to quit stressing to such an extent.

Acknowledge what it is that begins the stress.

Be explicit - if it's a particular occasion that triggers the tension, investigate it, record the subtleties if fundamental and get genuinely of the issue. For example, if it's financial problems, ensure that your outgoings don't surpass your salary. A suitable technique for watching out for your spending is to discount your use in two segments - "basics" and "extravagances." You will find that the last part will be twofold, treble, even ten times more than the previous. The genuine solaces of life cost not exactly many envision.

**Stress and dread.**

Ask yourself how often per day you fuss about something. Stress is lost vitality. It resembles an armchair, continues onward however never gets anyplace. It is a hopeless condition, making you and others close you miserable. Stop the propensity. How? By shaping new plans of work, play and articulation and living each day by itself. Make changes and begin once more. Mae West once said something like "you just live once, however When you do it right, once is sufficient."

**Get the upbeat propensity.**

Disentangle your day by day living, make some time for being calm, don't make your work or home your slave. Sleep, help somebody who is down; volunteer.

A decent exercise routine (indeed, I realize it's the old get fit prosaism) will help to concentrate the brain on different issues as opposed to always stressing over something that may never occur. Material prosperity has a noticeable impact on the soundness of the mind.

**Discussion about it.**

If you believe you can impart your worries to companions or family, you may find that you gain a new edge to your fears. When you would prefer not to converse with them, talk with your pet, at any rate, they won't contend with you.

Attempt to recollect - 1 - perceive your stress triggers, 2 - you can change how you live yet not your identity, and 3 - share your issues and make a move today.

The most effective method to Stop Worrying About SEO

There is one thing that you can depend on in Internet advertising. This is a new web index update each year. With the measure of individuals endeavoring to wind up tycoons medium-term in Internet advertising and attempting to trap the web crawlers, you are continually going to discover low-quality content and spam. This

The section will disclose to you what to do for the last time, not stress over SEO until kingdom come.

## 1. Quit Creating Bad Content

The most straightforward approach to quitting agonizing over SEO is to make great content from the begin. Concentrate on building up an association with your peruser first with your articles. At that point, stress over introducing an item and administration a short time later. Too often, Internet marketers stress over entering the subject and administration first without building up a relationship.

Consider how you like to be sold when you go to a disconnected store. Is it true that you usually are purchasing from the person that is attempting to stick an item under your throat that you know he's created the most cash? Or on the other hand, do you appreciate being sold to the person that needs to think about your needs and needs and build up an association with you?

In case you're the kind of person that preferences connections, present your online business along these lines also. Make educational articles, agreeable digital broadcast, and recordings that are enlightening to your perusers. These are the first things that your perusers are going to see, and they will build up the early introduction of you. Do it right, and you won't need to stress over extravagant direct mail advertisements or crush pages since the more significant part of the pre-selling has been done in your content.

## 2. Quit Trying to Manipulate the Search Engines

Let's be honest; Google is a vibrant organization that can contract loads and heaps of brilliant individuals to help make their web crawler calculations better. I don't think about you, yet it is highly unlikely that I'm more intelligent than a Harvard Ph.D. graduate, not to mention a thousand of them.

Spare yourself the time and disappointment on controlling the web search tools, as it'll never work long haul. Instead, center all your vitality around doing it directly in any case. Like this, when an update hits and you did things right, you will be compensated and not rebuffed.

Playing the passing by Google game is a specific flame method for winding up broke in the city. When Google makes sense of what everyone's doing; likewise, they make a fundamental change, and all that work has gone downhill. You can be rest ensured that they would rebuff you with every one of those additional backlinks that are exceptionally unimportant and it will cost you more in time and cash attempting to fix the issues than it would've when you did it effectively from the begin.

**The most effective method to Stop Worrying About What Other People Think**

For specific individuals, other individuals' suppositions don't make a difference. They can approach their day by day business while never addressing what other individuals may make of their activities, their decision of garments or what they said at the last workforce gathering. For other individuals, in any case, the constant stress over the conclusions of others can have an exceptionally negative effect on everyday life; taken to boundaries, it can turn out to be extraordinarily harmed.

It's normal to look for the endorsement of friends and family when we settle on choices or changes in our lives. Is it common, in any case, to toss a sweater you've worn once into the rubbish since somebody at the workplace says they're not very enthusiastic about the shading? The straightforward response to that question is no!

Low self-assurance can prompt us, putting an improper measure of significance on the assessments of other individuals. We're so uncertain of our capacities and convictions that we look to others when remarkably there's no compelling reason to. Stressing ceaselessly over other individuals' conclusions can be extremely destructive; it can likewise be a hard propensity to break. However, it tends to be finished. Here's the ticket:

**Self-acknowledgment**

Figure out how to acknowledge yourself for what you are. Advise yourself that you are a decent and minding individual and be cheerful that you are. Try not to put it all on the line attempting to be prominent; if you acknowledge yourself for your identity, anticipate that other individuals should do likewise.

**Grin**

At the point when certainty is low, it's anything but difficult to trust that individuals are deciding for you when in actuality, they aren't. Understand that individuals are excessively occupied with their very own lives and their very own issues to give much consideration to what you're doing.

If you do experience negative input from somebody, the best weapon in your arsenal is your grin. Whenever somebody says to you, "I truly don't care for that shading on you," grin sweetly and react with, "Well, I think what you're wearing is delightful." You'll be stunned at how great it makes you feel! At the point when individuals are terrible to us, and we don't react in the manner they foresee, it can genuinely toss them; sometimes enough to make them mull over disparaging remarks later on.

## Change your core interest

Figure out how to concentrate on what will satisfy you instead of taking a gander at what will persuade others. If something will meet you and you're not harming any other individual, feel free to do it. Understand that if other individuals can't be glad to see you having a good time, they're most likely not the sort of individuals you need to stick around with.

## Encircle yourself with inspiration

Investing energy with individuals who are negative or excessively basic can make you progressively slanted to look for endorsement consistently. Find a way to expel yourself from the impact of antagonistic individuals and decrease (if not stop out and out) the time you go through with them. You'll see that being around individuals who are additionally tolerating of you drives you to be all the more tolerating of yourself.

## Work towards raising your confidence

These different techniques will possibly work if you additionally do some chip away at your confidence. As you rest comfortable thinking about yourself, you will typically start to think less about what other individuals believe. Here two straightforward plans to kick you off:

## Set aside a few minutes for yourself

It's critical to require investment out from attempting to satisfy every other person and center around yourself for some time. Setting aside a few minutes for yourself is something that you should mean to do this regularly and permit yourself one rare treat every week. This is a viable method for advising yourself that you are an advantageous individual, and you have the right to do things that satisfy you. It may be something as basic as turning off the telephone and lying in an air pocket shower for 60 minutes. It could be meeting a companion to take a brief trip and see a motion picture. You could even get yourself a back rub or a new haircut. Whatever you pick, ensure it's about you and doesn't feel regretful; you merit it!

## Take up a new interest.

There are not many things as fulfilling as discovering something new that you adore and are great at. Taking up a new leisure activity is a fantastic method to chip away at your confidence. The fraternity with others and average premium can help to assemble certainty and understanding that you're learning new expertise and improving at something is a charming method to upgrade your confidence.

# CHAPTER FIVE
## Stress Relief and Guided Meditation

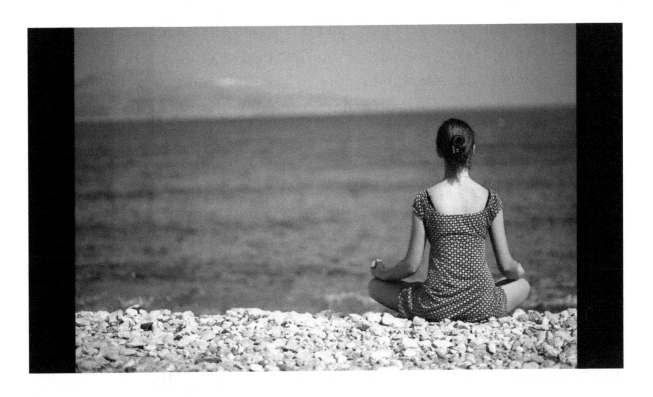

## You Are Being Nudged

You are being bumped each an everyday from your internal direction, and this is the thing that we call guided reflection. Stress alleviation and guided meditation are the points at which you focus on these prods, (which are signs), and you want to get some downtime. Feeling this guided reflection makes you feel increasingly associated because you usually are lead to inward smoothness. If you put the bumps off, the pushes will be industrious until you genuinely focus on them and take care of business. Taking care of this diligence may include contemplation, yet additionally, exercise and eating the correct sustenances. A great deal of the reasons we feel pushed is a direct result of the lifestyle we live in.

## Direction draws near...

Inside you, there is a bit of you pausing and needing quietness. This is a needing profound inside your soul, and it is frantically endeavoring to clear your pressure and bring you alleviation. The pushes are needing and subsequently are your internal direction. The mind produces considerations in your account again and again and likes to put you off track by putting you under a magnifying glass during reflection. The brain is willing you to diversion with sentiments like stress, uneasiness, and dread. Thinking is the point at which the mind calms; the body unwinds, the muscles relax, you are guided to quietness as your musings travel through you. Reflecting 15 minutes or more for every day will bring you stress help stunning.

## Envision Guidance and Meditation

Envision being guided elsewhere, similar to a field of wildflowers or the shoreline. You at that point start to feel the delicateness of your being and see how significant it is for your prosperity to envision. You become one with the minute, and it doesn't make a difference what you do in this creative mind since you're relinquishing this reality. Abandoning upsetting life occasions even only for a minute can have enduring impacts after. Envision...

## Tuning in After Meditation

It is critical to focus on what comes after you ruminate. It may not be immediately that you recognize what to do, yet the stresses you may have had before may not make any difference any longer. The pressure and the inquiries you had back will have answers that will come. Bit by bit as you become acclimated to reflection, you will see that the most significant piece of your day is contemplating and afterward focusing on signs.

# 4 Great Tips for Natural Anxiety Relief

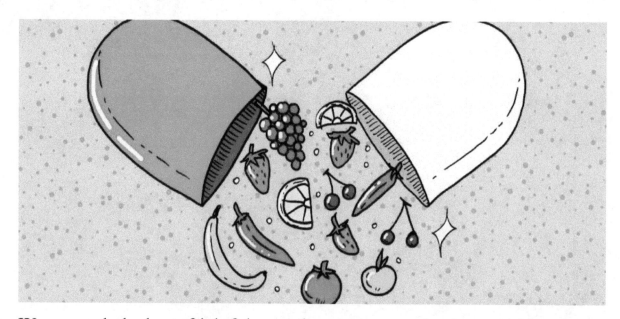

We, as a whole, have frightful, negative, counterproductive considerations now and then. However, the distinction between somebody who is inclined towards uneasiness and somebody who isn't is their main event with these considerations once they have them. Here we'll talk about a four-advance system you can figure out how to do whenever you need some quick, common nervousness help'. The ideal example of the restless individual is typically hugely unsurprising.

At the point when a restless idea armada into your mindfulness, you quickly respond with dread, a dread you can feel in your gut like you've been punched in the stomach. In light of the real response to the idea, you begin harping on the on edge though. Your body responds considerably more, which makes you start addressing yourself, "For what reason am I contemplating this? For what reason wouldn't I be able to stop? What's the issue with me? I believe I'm going insane, and I can't relax." And on it goes.

Here are essential fits of anxiety treatment that can help stop this endless loop before it begins.

## Stage One: Observe Your Thoughts

It appears to be irrational. However, you should give the negative considerations a chance to come in. The more agreeable you can be with them, the better. What you need to do is figure out how to change your response to them. What's more, by changing your answer to the musings, you become free of them.

When you can change your response to the considerations, would you be able to see it doesn't make a difference if you have them or not? It's your response that characterizes your existence. Everybody experiences negative temporary considerations. The thing that matters is the restless individual gets worked up about them, while others see them for what they are and disregard them. If you have ever reflected, you comprehend that you build up a tranquil personality, not by shutting out all idea, as though that were even conceivable! You understand that you have contemplations, so you let them float into your mindfulness and afterward pull out, merely seeing them. At the point when the on-edge individual has a negative idea, they ought to do precisely the equivalent. To begin with, watch it, as though you were a fair eyewitness. Notice that you are reconsidering that.

## Stage Two: Name Your Thoughts

At that point, name your negative considerations. "Truly, that is my old friend - fill in the clear." Some regular names for reviews would be "social nervousness" or "dread of driving off an extension."

**Stage Three: Watch Your Thoughts**

At that point watch the idea go, without judging. Try not to begin getting into the endless loop of contrary reasoning which heightens your tension.

**Stage Four: Move On**

At that point, move your consideration on to what you are doing. Try not to attempt to drive the idea to leave, either. That resembles the old joke, "don't consider a pink elephant," and that turns into everything you can consider! So, to total up this uneasiness cure, first, you watch, name, listen, at that point move on. Of course, this isn't the primary usual nervousness treatment that has worked for other people. This is a champion among the essential types of uneasiness self-improvement, and you can start to utilize it today. It will take some training. This is an incredible system. However, you may want a more extensive, organized program that can direct you and keep you concentrated on what you have to do to take out your uneasiness and frenzy manifestations effectively.

# Stress and Anxiety Relief - Three Helpful Techniques

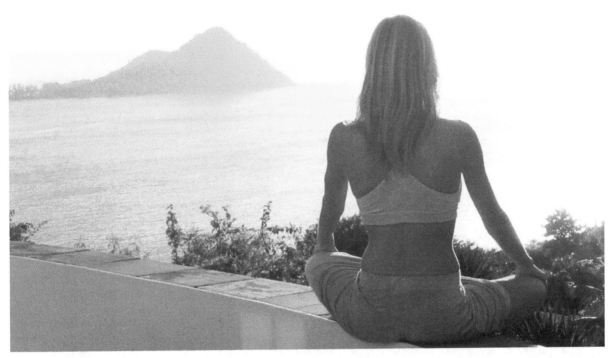

You are feeling pushed and overpowered, and you need some pressure alleviation! On occasion, we as a whole do need pressure help as there are certain circumstances and conditions where we could genuinely utilize this alleviation. At the point when our dimensions of physical, mental, and enthusiastic strain are overpowering us, we are in all respects liable to learn about pushed. This can be harming to our wellbeing, our connections, our profession, and all aspects of our life. Before you even get to that point, let's talk about specific tips to enable you to deal with your worry for those days that are overpowering:

## 1. Mindfulness Meditation

Mindfulness reflection is as a rule occupied with the present minute. As indicated by a UW-Madison research group, there was an expansion of enactment in the left-side piece of the frontal locale. This recommends reflection itself creates more significant movement in this locale of the mind which is related to lower tension and a progressively positive enthusiastic state. In this manner, mindfulness reflection can genuinely change how the cerebrum processes things and can fortify the regions of the mind related to bringing down pressure. Without learning of this investigation, I have seen this to be valid in myself, just as the majority of my customers that are currently doing mindfulness reflection. It's completely astonishing!

## 2. Perception

Our psyches are ground-breaking!! Representation, which is additionally called guided symbolism, is regularly to some reflection systems for reconstructing our psychological states. When we envision ourselves in a tranquil scene, you can take advantage of those sentiments of being quiet and genuinely figure out how to feel this serene inclination all the more regularly in your everyday life in spite of what might occur around you. Envision, truly observe and feel yourself in that spot that presents to you a grin and harmony. Close your eyes and attempt it now. Experience how it feels and appreciates it. That mind split far from your stressors is a decent get-away for your cerebrum. Appreciate!

## 3. Extend

At the point when the body is feeling focused on, it is regularly tight and tense. Frequently when working with individuals to discharge pressure, specialists of different types, all-encompassing and customary, will primarily work with the psyche and passionate procedures. While these are helpful and do work very well when polished, so does working out our worry through the body. Set aside some effort to stretch out your muscles, your legs, your neck, you bear, your back, and the remainder of your body. When you do as such, appreciate the stretch and recollect to breathe.

Attempt these pressure alleviation tips before you get overpowered, so you don't get to that point where you need to rip your hair out! On the off chance that you are by then officially, at that point, do this NOW!

**Would meditation be able to Help You Reduce Anxiety?**

If you are gotten up to speed in the cycle of pressure and tension to the point you are encountering fits of anxiety, is it conceivable you can discover alleviation in something as straightforward as contemplation? It is anything but difficult to reject reflection as new age gibberish. However, we should take a second and look at it all the more intently.

Stress and tension can trigger your bodies' battle or flight instruments. It expands your adrenaline. You experience short, shallow relaxing. Your heart pulsates quicker. Your muscles worry as though you are getting ready for a physical blow.

Contemplation, in its most comfortable structure, is moderately loosened up relaxing. Deep moderate breathing can bring down your pulse. It can assist you with relaxing your muscles. The principal objective of reflection is to clear your psyche of unpleasant considerations as well as of all suspected.

So, when you consider it, reflection is gone for delivering the careful inverse impact on your body as pressure.

Reflection is gone for creating a condition of profound quiet and serenity, which enables you to clear your brain of upsetting considerations and feelings. It can likewise help improve specific ailments.

Contemplation has been around for a great many years. While a few people like to concentrate on the profound angles, it's anything but essential for encountering the physical advantages.

If you are keen on trying different things with reflection the incredible thing about it is all you need is 5-20 minutes of available time and when you are a first beginning, a pleasant calm spot to sit. As you become progressively gifted at the reflection, you will find that you can rehearse it anyplace.

Contemplation can take on various structures. There is guided reflection where you center around visual pictures of spots and circumstances you find unwinding. There is mantra contemplation which spotlights on utilizing a word or expression to take out diverting musings. There is careful reflection where the objective is to figure out how to live more at the time.

If none of these styles advance to you, at that point there are kinds of reflection that include physical development and are gone for clearing the brain, for example, Qi Gong, Tai Chi, and Yoga.

When stress and tension have surpassed you when fits of anxiety are restricting your capacity to have a glad existence, would you be able to stand to neglect any road of conceivable treatment? Possibly reflection can enable you to mitigate pressure and decrease your uneasiness. Take a full breath out it an attempt!

# Step by step instructions to Cope with Anxiety Naturally

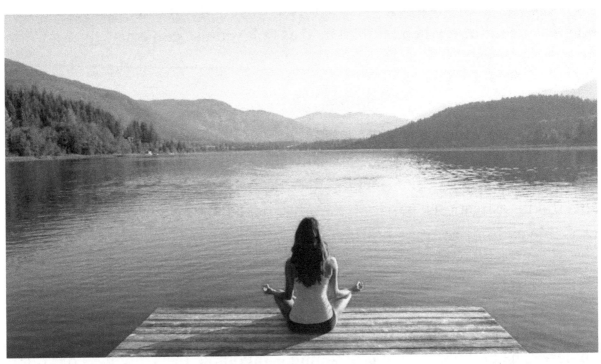

Nervousness is a sentiment of dread, stress, or anxiety. It can influence your activities, considerations, emotions, and even your physical wellbeing. When you are one of the large numbers of individuals who experience the ill effects of uneasiness consistently, read on to find unique approaches to adapt to this condition.

**Homegrown Remedies for Anxiety**

Many herbs can be valuable in helping you manage nervousness. Following is a rundown of herbs that may ease explicit side effects of uneasiness usually:

**Kava -** This herb has been demonstrated to be exceptionally compelling in the treatment of tension. It is a pressure reducer and muscle relaxant. Care ought to be utilized when taking kava, as delayed use can cause liver harm.

**Passionflower -** Drink this herb in tea structure to quiet your nerves. Passionflower will lessen pressure and loosen up your muscles. It can likewise be utilized to treat other typical side effects of uneasiness, for example, cerebral pains, a sleeping disorder, and emotional episodes. In specific investigations, passionflower has been demonstrated to be similarly as viable as some solution hostile to uneasiness drugs.

**Chamomile -** This mainstream herb can help treat most side effects of tension. It is viable in the treatment of sleep deprivation, migraines, and anxiety. The best part is that chamomile is favorable the soundness of your liver and lungs.

**Valerian -** Valerian is an extraordinary regular narcotic. It can enable you to get a decent night's rest and can be utilized to treat mellow uneasiness. This ought not to be blended with another enemy of nervousness medicates or used by kids under 12.

**Bounces -** This natural cure can be utilized for the treatment of every single real side effect of uneasiness. It is an incredible decision for facilitating cerebral pains, quieting your nerves, and to use as a narcotic. The surprising thing about bounces is that there are no known symptoms. Bounces have numerous other medical advantages like the capacity to lessen fevers and treat skin diseases.

## Unwinding Techniques to Ease Anxiety

Contemplation is an excellent method to quiet your body and psyche. There is a wide range of techniques for consideration that you can use to help hold your uneasiness under control. Practically these strategies include controlled breathing and loosening up your body.

To begin, you have to locate an agreeable spot and sit or lay in a usually loosened up position (you don't have to sit with folded legs). Close your eyes and take in for a tally of 3, hold this breath for a score of 3, and afterward discharge it gradually for a check of 3. Focus on your relaxing for a couple of minutes until it winds up characteristic. Presently get the chance to deal with loosening up your brain. Some think that its more straightforward to focus on one picture, while others endeavor to clear their psyches of everything. If you are merely starting, it is most likely more straightforward to focus on a specific something.

If you find that it is difficult to think, you may think about guided reflection or even trance. You can discover recordings on the web that will walk you through observation well ordered.

## Exercise Reduces Anxiety and Stress

Practicing is significant for the general prosperity of anybody. In any case, it is significantly progressively significant for sufferers of tension. Doing cardiovascular activities all the time will support your dissemination. This implies more oxygen is being conveyed all through your body and your cerebrum. This, by itself, can soothe cerebral pains and stress. Another extraordinary favorable position to practicing is that it discharges endorphins in your mind. These endorphins will give you a general feeling of prosperity. If you start practicing consistently, you will, without a doubt, see that sentiments of nervousness will be less successive.

# Does Thinking Positively Make a Difference?

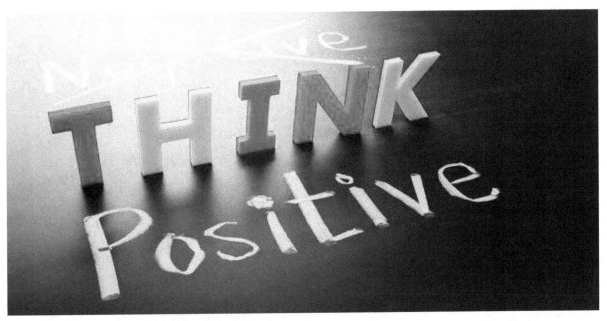

If you have been feeling down, there is a valid justification for why it is going on. It may be the case that you are experiencing a tough time in your life, or it may be the case that you are discouraged. Discouragement is something that strikes many individuals; however, they once in a while, comprehend that they have an ailment. Regardless of why you are down when you are discouraged for over about fourteen days with no real-life occasion causing that feeling, see your specialist about despondency. You can take drugs to feel much improved, and you can likewise find out about the intensity of reasoning entirely.

Regardless of what somebody lets you know, you cannot simply snap out of melancholy. It isn't that basic. Those that state that doesn't comprehend what sadness truly is. There is something to said for working with your specialist on prescriptions and endeavoring to work out an approach to begin thinking decidedly. It's anything but a supernatural occurrence fix and not in every case simple, yet it very well may be something you do that causes you to turn your life around. Indeed, even those that are not discouraged can take in something from positive reasoning all through life when things are great and when things are terrible.

There is no exact science behind the thought, yet some feel that only thinking decidedly can transform yourself around. The inclination is that if you accept that things will turn out badly, they will and that when you expect that things will go well, they will. The power is in the reasoning and in what you do with the emotions that your thinking achieves. If you are thinking positively, you will do the correct things for that positive result. Then again, you could likewise do the wrong things when thinking negative contemplations. Most don't realize they are doing it, yet it might be precisely what's going on.

Although you cannot by any stretch of the imagination trust that when you need something awful enough you can have it, or the world would be brimming with only specialists, demigods, entertainers, presidents, ballet performers, firefighters, and proficient competitors. You can buckle down and put your everything towards something and not get it. In any case, pondering what you need and progressing in the direction of its ups your odds of making your fantasies work out as expected. You can apply this to any part of your life, and you may get what you need. If not, it may be the case that reasoning emphatically opens entryways you were not expecting, and you will finish up in a far better spot.

Have a go at speculation decidedly in your life in little things and see what occurs. You cannot be sure that you are going to win a million when you scratch off a lottery ticket. However, you can feel that your new higher education is going to enable you to get your fantasy work. When your tyke is having issues, think in a positive way that you are going to support them. Your positive contemplations can enable you to locate the correct arrangement. If you don't know what to do at work when an issue emerges, you are thinking positively may help. You get the thought. Check whether it doesn't work for you.

# 7 Easy Steps to Think Positive and Change Your Life

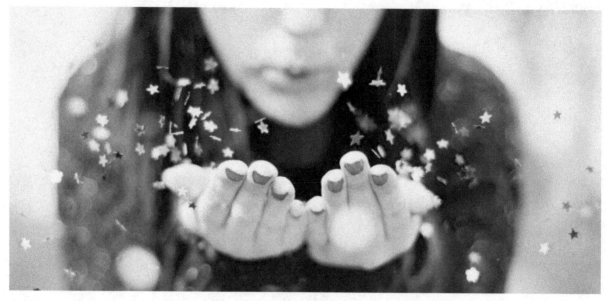

Positive reasoning can add such a significant amount to your life - and now we realize that positive thinking can add a long time to your life. When you think positive, you dispose of pressure and will, in general, carry on with more useful life and settle on better decisions. In case you're usually a negative mastermind, there are ways you can change that reasoning and jump on the way to life getting updated perspective.

If you genuinely need to start to think definitely and transform yourself to improve things, take a gander at the accompanying advances you can join into your way of life:

1. Be in charge of your musings. Nobody can reveal to you what to think or controls how you respond to your reasoning. When you start to assume liability for your considerations, you'll face the truth of what they're doing to or for you and be progressively ready to change those negative musings.

2. Plan to think decidedly. So many of our considerations originate from the subliminal personality. When you intend to believe unquestionably, you won't be as well-suited to take what you suppose as the real world. Instead, you have room schedule-wise and chance to thoroughly consider it and arrive at the resolution that mirrors the truth.

3. Stay away from pessimistic individuals. Pessimistic individuals can destroy your best-laid designs to think decidedly. They can bolster the flame of self-uncertainty and tension. It can now and again be delegated a group attitude, so don't fall prey to it. Have an independent perspective.

4. Record your contemplations. It's useful if you can see by the day's end what your considerations have been. For a moment, set aside the effort to record them. You'll see what turned out badly with your contemplations and have the option to improve them.

5. Think about the repercussions. For instance, if you have a due date for a task and it turns out to be evident that you're not going to meet it, think about what may occur. If you complete it on schedule, it won't be in the same class as you needed. In the fact that you take additional time, it might cause different issues. Additionally, think about the arrangements. For instance, you could request an augmentation to the due date.

6. Limit calamitous reasoning. As opposed to contemplating a circumstance, attempt to limit it, and lower your uneasiness level by being handy about it. In case you're vulnerable to those considerations, dodge circumstances, (for example, TV news) that my reason for restless reasoning.

7. Live for the occasion. When you contribute an additional measure of vitality attempting to figure or break down the future, you'll persuade yourself regarding disappointment - mainly when you've bombed before. If you think you'll come up short, you likely will.

Acknowledge the truth that you can control your considerations. You'll turn out to be progressively enabled to confront distressing circumstances throughout your life and to change how you think. It will end up more straightforward to keep up an uplifting disposition the more you work on intuition decidedly.

When you need an existence without uncertainty and dread and where neither nervousness nor enthusiastic irregularity is influencing your life's results; where your life is giving you:

- Complete equalization and congruity in your affection, life, and your expert life.

- Enthusiastic Freedom to feel settled, quiet, and in control, grasping your identity.

- Asserting and owning your capacity and;

- Accepting and confiding in a future where you feel boundless in what you can accomplish.

- Instructions to Think Positive Thoughts

- Instructions to think positive considerations that is the unavoidable issue!

Each idea we have isn't always solid and centered. The most significant piece of our day is depleted or spent in supposed minor musings, which are temporary contemplations that come and go and for the most part, does not help us in being sure.

Different sorts of contemplations that are not pretty much nothing or brief accumulate around comparative considerations. They are altogether joined around similar subjects and made convictions.

We can create our musings, or we can receive them from others. A portion of our contemplations was assembled all through our adolescence.

These considerations were in a general sense, not our own. We acquired them from our mom and father, family, and later from educators or potentially religious pioneers.

Furthermore, presently let's verify how these two gatherings of thought can make an impact on our life.

## 1-Big musings or convictions

If a couple of considerations are gathering around a similar idea and shaping a conviction, at that point, those contemplations are loaded up with a critical enthusiastic charge. These considerations will pull in your regular day to day existence similar individuals and conditions that offer the same vitality.

We make our world through our contact with the high intensity of free will.

When our convictions are sure, they will present to us some goals to every one of the difficulties that we are looked with during the most poorly designed conditions.

Having contemplations of overall achievement joined with an uplifting standpoint will carry you to a real existence brimming with parity and concordance.

Any place we go, regardless of whether we change the country we live in, our musings remain with us. Our convictions are always bringing into our lives, similar conditions, and occasions.

The fundamental issue that the majority of us battle with ordinary are negative contemplations and Ideas, which we animate by having confidence in them.

Ideally, you presently see how much harm you can do to yourself as well as other people in your surroundings by not having a decent inspirational standpoint.

Along these lines, you can and will pull in negative impacts into your life and not understand that you are doing it. By not being sure, you will influence everybody and everything in your life.

## 2-Small musings

Little transient negative considerations that can incidentally fly through your conscious personality and similarly as fast fly away could deliver awful states of mind, and complicated emotions, without knowing why or the logical reasoning behind it.

The issue with little contemplations coming all through your cognizant personality is that they as a rule return, and each time they do sadly can get more grounded and all the more persuading. All things considered, 70 percent of people group's contemplations are pessimistic from the everyday.

Delight throughout everyday life and your inward vitality are stolen ordinary when you think negatively.

Showing and developing into new convictions is actually what minor negative contemplations can do whenever left unchecked. This could draw in progressively negative things or occasions into your life.

The opportunity of decision is in our grasp. If you embed the idea and trust that ordinary you draw in what you think, we can make supernatural occurrences in our lives and improve it definitely by deduction positive.

In that manner, we can find two critical exercises which are an ordinary good faith and a presence brimming with bliss.

When you open your eyes, you will see the Law of Attraction is working surrounding you. In your life, in your connections, in your work environment, you can draw in everything that you need.

**You need to consider what you truly need.**

Your considerations can show your life into a physical reality. Try not to slight all that you have perused here or the essential standards we have talked about here. Do your best not to settle on a poor decision.

As a rule in life, we don't understand or comprehend certain things that occur in our life; however, we once in a while use them to support ourselves. By figuring out how to think positive musings and by associating that with being sure in our regular day to day existence, we would all be able to make elevating contemplations to move ourselves as well as other people near us.

# CONCLUSION

Most by far of us have had the experience of inclination inconceivably constructive about an occasion, an individual, or a result we have buckled down for, yet regularly that feeling doesn't last. As time turns into a memory, so does the positive inclination. You may review that as a kid, you may get up every morning liking nothing specifically, for reasons unknown by any stretch of the imagination. Envision having the option to do that consistently for an incredible reminder. So, when we have coincidentally adapted some idea designs that make us hopeless in either a specific situation or life when all is said in done, how would we approach transforming them to a more 'think positive' approach?

Three fundamental conditions need to exist first: You should be so tired of inclination terrible, down, harmful, and so on that, you choose you genuinely need to transform; You need to see the issue of disposition negative from another point of view; You should discover or make new and engaging alternatives.

When you make for yourself the decision of a positive change, you are bound to pick the positive alternative than the negative ones.

You could begin by asking yourself: "Would I like to encounter my first day of inclination amazingly constructive for reasons unknown specifically today or tomorrow?" and "Would I like to feel constructive all in all or about a specific occasion or individual?"

To retune your cerebrum to be increasingly positive, complete this activity:

Unwind and inhale profoundly, and as you unwind, it winds up simpler and more straightforward to give your creative mind a chance to play. Presently envision another you, remaining before you, this is the most magnificently positive, feeling useful for reasons unknown by any stretch of the imagination, you, that you can envision - your real positive self. Set aside some effort to contact content with the positive you, see how the positive you stand, grins, inhales, talks, moves. Notice how energy emanates like shining light from the positive you, see how the positive you handle issues and accomplishes objectives. Presently transform the positive you around and venture into and coordinate with your credible positive self. Transparent the eyes of your positive person, hear through the ears of your positive and feel how incredible inclination positive feels. Invest some energy staring off into space about how your life will improve as your life increasingly more as your positive real self.


Numerous individuals think that it's painful to finish the activity first thing on a morning before getting up or the last word during the evening (don't attempt the event while driving or working hardware). You can utilize this activity as a significant aspect of your general improvement or when you need an additional shot of that 'think positive' demeanor.

CPSIA information can be obtained
at www.ICGtesting.com
Printed in the USA
LVHW010817010621
689026LV00011B/1303